W9-DEA-047

The Gigantic Book of Running Quotations

The Gigantic Book of Running Quotations

Edited and Introduced by Hal Higdon

Foreword by Amby Burfoot

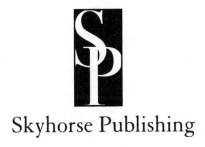

Skyhorse Publishing

Skyhorse Publishing books may be purchased in bulk at special discounts for sales promotion, corporate gifts, fund raising, or educational purposes. Special editions can also be created to specifications. For details, contact Special Sales Department, Skyhorse Publishing, 555 Eighth Avenue, Suite 903, New York, NY 10018 or info@skyhorsepublishing.com.

www.skyhorsepublishing.com

Library of Congress Cataloging-in-Publication Data

Higdon, Hal.
The gigantic book of running quotations / edited and introduced by Hal Higdon; foreword by Amby Burfoot.
    p. cm.
 ISBN 978-1-60239-251-9 (hardcover : alk. paper) 1. Running—Quotations, maxims, etc. 2. Running—Miscellanea. I. Title.

GV1061.M39 2008
796.42—dc22

                                         2007050710

10 9 8 7 6 5 4 3 2 1

Printed in the United States of America

Contents

Foreword

I've long believed that many runners have the wrong idea about what it takes to succeed in the mile, the 10K, cross-country, the marathon, or whatever your chosen distance might be. You don't need long legs. You don't need a skinny frame. You don't need a special diet or a secret training plan. You don't even need an over-sized heart capable of pumping vast quantities of oxygen-rich blood to all parts of your body. (Though that's a good thing, no doubt about it.)

What you need is motivation, and lots of it. Enough motivation to stick to a consistent running program. Because without consistency, none of the above (not even a big heart) will improve your performances.

The best motivation comes from a steadfast friend (or many such friends). A literal friend and training partner is a great asset, but not always available. A second option and a constant, always-there-when-you-need-him/her friend is the inspirational running quote. Too stressed by work deadlines to fit in your run? Reach for a great quote. Too fatigued by family responsibilities? A little quote will do you. Too sleepy to get out of bed for your morning run? Make sure you've got a favorite quote close at hand.

I know few lifelong runners who don't have dozens of favorite running quotes—from the Bible, from Shakespeare, from other poets, from songs, from famous leaders, from philosophers, and from many other sources. We post these quotes in all our most important life spaces—at home, at work, in training logs, on calendars, and of course on the refrigerator, where they often battle for space with prized photos of families and friends. We feel lost and somewhat vulnerable if we look around and don't spot one of our revered quotes. We recognized their power; we want to keep them close to us.

I readily recall the key moments of my own evolution as a quote fan. When I was young, like all children, I had a favorite book that I begged my parents to read over and over again. It was *The Little Engine That Could*, the story of the tiny locomotive that achieved what bigger rivals couldn't simply by repeating "I think I can, I think I can" over and over again. Many decades later, I'm somewhat embarrassed to admit how much this simplistic tale meant to me. Somewhat. But not totally. In fact, I expect *The Little Engine* had more influence on my life than I've ever fully realized.

In junior high, I read dozens of books in the "Chip Hilton" sports series, and there I first encountered the old chestnut, "When the going gets tough, the tough get going." Again, it's ridiculously simple. But also a bit catchy. And I've probably used this quote more often than any other when I needed a burst of extra energy in a tough race or workout.

The older I got, the more great quotes I encountered, and the more diverse. Some from great thinkers, some from fast and famous runners, and some from writers who had a delightfully skewed perspective on life. In my lexicon, the quote both humorous and motivational is a special treasure. I particularly enjoy a number of Lewis Carroll quotes. When I'm on a treadmill, I always think about this observation from the Red Queen: "It takes all the running you can do to keep in the same place. If you want to get somewhere else, you must run at least twice as fast." Now, I know that doesn't sound encouraging, but it always brings a smile to my face, and the smile helps me run smoother.

When daunted by a difficult task, I like to remember one of Alice's conversations from *Alice in Wonderland*. Alice protests the futility of trying to believe in the impossible. But the Queen retorts that Alice obviously hasn't tried very hard, noting, "Why, sometimes I've believed as many as six impossible things before breakfast." Personally, at that early an hour, I'm usually willing to settle for just one or two.

I'll mention just two more favorite quotes. As a runner who has spent forty years striving to stay both fit and competitive, I've always been drawn to the words of 1989 New York City Marathon champion Juma Ikangaa. Ikangaa, a Tanzanian who raced frequently in the United States, once said: "The will to win means nothing without the will to prepare." This quote will get me out of bed almost any morning, no matter now dark and dreary.

Finally, here's my favorite running quote among all the thousands that you'll find on the pages that follow. It comes from the writings of Dr. George Sheehan, longtime *Runner's World* contributor, who probably coined more memorable and inspirational running phrases than any other author. Anytime you need a boost, Sheehan is sure to provide. The quote: "There are as many reasons for running as there are days in the year, years in my life. I run because I am an animal and a child, an artist and a saint."

I treasure this quote because I believe, as Wordsworth did, that we all contain multitudes. And that we are capable of finding many reasons for our runs—competitive reasons, health reasons, creative reasons, psychological reasons, spiritual reasons. Indeed, we run one day for one purpose, and another day with a completely different goal.

And for each of those goals, we can find a different quote to get us going. Enjoy them all. And treasure every run.

Amby Burfoot
January 2008

Introduction

In *Through the Looking Glass*, Lewis Carroll puts these words in the Red Queen's mouth: "Now, here, you see, it takes all the running you can do to keep in the same place. If you want to get somewhere else, you must run at least twice as fast as that."

Carroll's classic sequel to *Alice in Wonderland* was published in 1871, a full century before Jim Fixx's *The Complete Book of Running* sold a million copies in hardback and helped launch the running boom. But Carroll was hardly the first writer to tie a phrase to running. "Now bid me run," wrote William Shakespeare, "and I will strive with things impossible." The bard of Avon gave that line to Julius Caeser, though no evidence exists that Caeser ever ran a marathon. Come to think of it, the tale of Pheidippides running from the plains of Marathon into Athens, the legend we base our sport upon, owes more to fiction than to fact.

You will encounter the words of Carroll and Shakespeare in this seminal volume of *Running Wisdom*, compiled from many sources, but you also can enjoy the words of Burfoot, Henderson, Sheehan and Fixx. And a few quotes from Higdon too. As running has matured from boom to a defining movement that has shaped lives, new writers have emerged to stand on the slender shoulders of Amby, Joe, George, Jim and I. Kenny Moore, Tom Derderian and Roger Robinson for example. Olympic champions Emil Zatopek, Frank Shorter and Joan Benoit Samuelson have proved quotable. Their chosen words help enrich the pages of this book of running wisdom.

Lewis Carroll and William Shakespeare to the contrary, it seems that the recording of running bon mots began to thrive in the 1960s, a decade both dark with despair and bright with hope, an era when the Boston Marathon attracted only a few hundred starters, most of them capable of breaking 3 hours. I cashed my first paychecks as a magazine editor, then morphed into a freelance writer, embracing the freeness of that discipline partly because it gave me time to run in daylight. During my early career, I wrote about anything other than long distance running, because who wanted to read about that sport back in 1959?

That was the year I ran my first Boston. We were a scurvy lot, the 150 of us who showed up in Hopkinton, our deeds largely unheralded. And certainly there was little advice offered to those who wanted to conquer the marathon.

That soon would change. In 1966, a high school runner from Kansas named Bob Anderson started what was little more than a newsletter, called *Distance Running News*. It grew in circulation, so three years later Anderson dropped out of college and moved to California, hiring a young staffer from *Track & Field News* named Joe Henderson as editor. They changed the publication's name to *Runner's World* in time for the January 1970 issue, the first issue of the decade when running finally captured the interest of a public that previously assumed running to be a sport confined to the young and restless.

Many who would shape the world of running as we view it today came together about that time. Hopkinton Green, starting point for the Boston

Marathon, offered the common meeting ground. Dr. Kenneth Cooper, author of *Aerobics*, ran there in the early 1960s. So did Erich Segal, author of *Love Story*. Henderson first ran Boston in 1967. In 1968, Amby Burfoot, who one day would become editor of *Runner's World*, won the Boston Marathon. That same year and at the Olympic Games in Mexico City, I introduced Joe Henderson to a doctor friend and Boston fellow traveler: George Sheehan. Recruited by Joe, George would go on to become *Runner's World's* most popular columnist as well as a best-selling author. In 1971, I wrote a book titled *On The Run From Dogs and People*, its title borrowed from an article previously published by *Sports Illustrated*. Somewhat of a cult classic, that book remains in print today and provides at least one quote for this book.

All those named above contributed to the growth of a sport that eventually would be accepted by the masses, both those running marathons and watching them. Frank Shorter won the Olympic Marathon in 1972 and after that came Jim Fixx, and in the three decades following a host of running writers quoted in the pages following. They provide us with words of running wisdom.

Use these words as your inspiration and you will be able, as suggested by William Shakespeare, to strive with things impossible. You might even run fast enough to please Lewis Carroll.

—*Hal Higdon*
Contributing Editor:
Runner's World

CHAPTER ONE

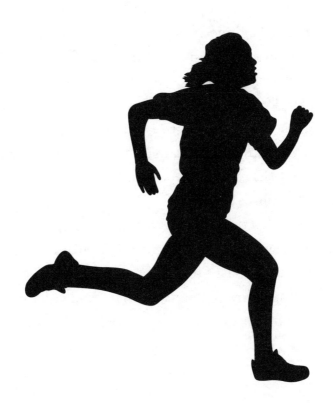

Ready to run?

Starting Line

The most important task for the beginning runner is that you "begin." A simple verb, full of sound and fury, signifying much, to paraphrase Shakespeare. Beginning is a chore most difficult to achieve. Unless you take that first step as a beginner, you are not going anywhere.

But so many individuals have put that first foot forward, taking a first step, even if it is not a running step. They follow with a second step, and this opens a world of hope. Soon a short stroll becomes a longer walk. A short jog becomes a longer run. Then one day you look up and find yourself on the starting line of a marathon surrounded by tens of thousands of individuals who, like you, might have taken their first running steps only months before.

Running comes with a price. Between that first step as a walker or a runner and steps taken during the 26 miles 385 yards of a marathon come moments of pleasure and—let's be honest—moments of pain.

But that goes with the joy of being a runner. And you cannot become a runner unless you first begin. A simple verb, full of sound and fury, leading to a lifetime commitment.

The world is divided into two kinds of people: runners and non-runners.

— MARC BLOOM, *THE RUNNER'S BIBLE*

———◦———

In a world that's quickly becoming so fast-paced that multi-tasking is a way of life, runners have managed to find a way to do something that's good for our heads, bodies, and spirits, and that provides wonderful social interaction.

— JOHN BINGHAM

———◦———

If walking upright first set early human ancestors apart from their ape cousins, it may have been their eventual ability to run long distances with a springing step over the African savanna that influenced the transition to today's human body form. . .

— JOHN NOBLE WILFORD, "RUNNING EXTRA MILES SETS THE HUMAN APART," *THE NEW YORK TIMES,* NOVEMBER 18, 2004

———◦———

Laziness is nothing more than the habit of resting before you get tired.

— JULES RENARD

Number one is just to gain a passion for running. To love the morning, to love the trail, to love the pace on the track. And if some kid gets really good at it, that's cool too.

— PAT TYSON

Running removes us briefly from the fragmentation and depersonalization of the digital world.

— AMBY BURFOOT, *THE RUNNER'S GUIDE TO THE MEANING OF LIFE*

I can't remember what I was doing before running. I guess shopping, sewing, watching TV—gaining nothing.

— MIKI GORMAN

———◆———

I'm afraid the reason so many new runners quit is because they never get past the point of feeling like they have to run.

— JOHN BINGHAM, "WHO NEEDS A REASON?" *RUNNERS WORLD*

———◆———

All runners, at one time or another, are beginners.

— *THE NEW YORK ROAD RUNNERS CLUB COMPLETE BOOK OF RUNNING*

———◆———

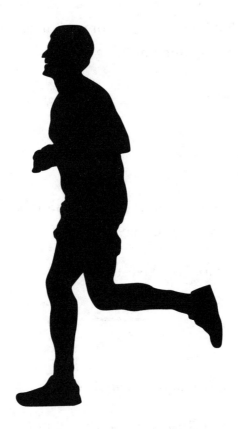

It is not so much that I began to run, but that I continued.

— HAL HIGDON

Now bid me run,
And I will strive with things impossible,
Yea, get the better of them.

— SHAKESPEARE, *JULIUS CAESAR*

A runner is real when she takes the first step.

— CLARISSA PINKOLA ESTÉS, PH.D.

Running is a great investment. Your principal is low. Your rate of return is enormous, and it keeps growing every year. And there are no hidden charges, unless you count an occasional blister.

— FLORENCE GRIFFITH JOYNER AND JON HANC, *RUNNING FOR DUMMIES*

Running is elementary. It is elegant in its simplicity.

— JOHN BINGHAM, *THE COURAGE TO START*

Just as you write down other important appointments, you need to literally pencil in time for your run. The process itself is empowering. In the few seconds it takes to scribble "run" into a time slot, you make running a part of your life.

— JEFF GALLOWAY

I'm not saying running could solve all of the world's problems, but I think it would be a good start.

— JOHN BINGHAM

Play is where life lives.

— GEORGE SHEEHAN

We may train or peak for a certain race, but running is a lifetime sport.

— ALBERTO SALAZAR

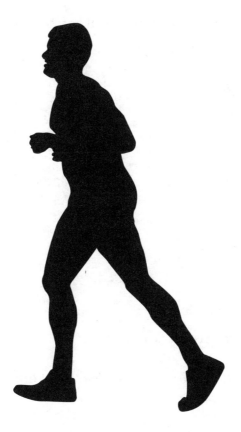

If you feel great the first day, like a million dollars, you're an exception.

— Marc Bloom

If you want to become the best runner you can be, start now. Don't spend the rest of your life wondering if you can do it.

— PRISCILLA WELCH

Endurance? You've only got to get out there and do it. Face up to it: Man was meant to run.

— PERCY CERUTTY

Running is not just exercise; it is a lifestyle.

— JOHN BINGHAM, *RUNNING FOR MORTALS: A COMMONSENSE PLAN FOR CHANGING YOUR LIFE WITH RUNNING*

I put it in historical perspective. This is our heritage; our evolutionary gift, dating back to our days as hunters and gatherers.

— STU MITTLEMAN

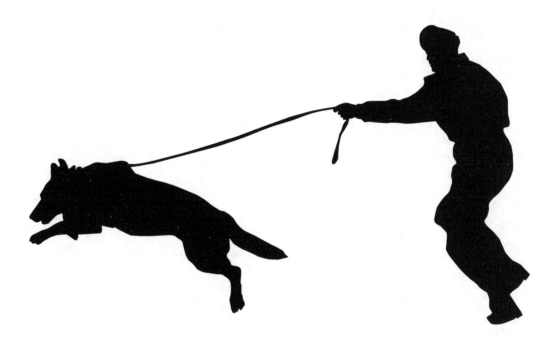

The most important message I stress to beginners is to learn to love the sport. Like other endeavors, if running is not undertaken properly, it can be difficult and discouraging.

— CLIFF HELD

A lot of people say they love running because of how they feel afterward. Not me. Well, I love that, too, but it's also so much fun while I'm out there.

— DICK BEARDSLEY

In the beginning you likely say, "I run." With more confidence, you say, "I am a runner."

— GLORIA AVERBUCH

[Y]ou were born to run. Maybe not that fast, maybe not that far, maybe not as efficiently as others. But to get up and move, to fire up that entire energy-producing, oxygen-delivering, bone-strengthening process we call running.

— FLORENCE GRIFFITH JOYNER AND JON HANC, *RUNNING FOR DUMMIES*

Now, here, you see, it takes all the running you can do, to keep in the same place. If you want to get somewhere else, you must run at least twice as fast as that.

— LEWIS CARROLL, *THROUGH THE LOOKING-GLASS*

———◆———

When people ask me why I run, I tell them, there's not really a reason, it's just the adrenaline when you start, and the feeling when you cross that finish line, and know that you are a winner no matter what place you got.

— COURTNEY PARSONS

———◆———

Running is a thing worth doing not because of the future rewards it bestows, but because of how it feeds our bodies and minds and souls in the present.

— KEVIN NELSON, *THE RUNNER'S BOOK OF DAILY INSPIRATION*

———◆———

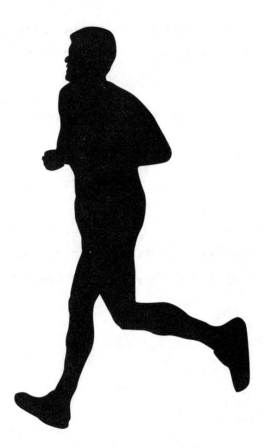

[Newly chosen kings went on a ceremonial run that] symbolized laying claim to his domain and proved that he was fit enough for the demands of his position.

— HISTORIAN EDWARD SEARS ON THE PRACTICE OF ANCIENT
    EGYPTIAN KINGS

For me, running is a lifestyle and an art. I'm more interested in the magic of it than the mechanics.

— LORRAINE MOLLER, FOUR-TIME NEW ZEALAND OLYMPIAN

Running is real and relatively simple—but it ain't easy.

— MARK WILL-WEBER

Every time I walk out the door, I know why I'm going where I'm going and I'm already focused on that special place where I find my peace and solitude.

— SASHA AZEVEDO

The advice I have for beginners is the same philosophy that I have for runners of all levels of experience and ability—consistency, a sane approach, moderation and making your running an enjoyable, rather than dreaded, part of your life.

— *BILL RODGERS' LIFETIME RUNNING PLAN*

Starting is scary. It is for everyone. . . . I never allowed my eyes to meet those of other runners, because I was afraid of seeming like an impostor.

— JOHN BINGHAM, *THE COURAGE TO START*

Do something that involves use of the body. How can you hope to run when you spend the whole day standing still? How can you hope to master your own body when your body is the slave of a machine?

— BRIAN GANVILLE, "THE OLYMPIAN"

If someone could find a way to bottle motivation, he would make a fortune.

— HAL HIGDON

It's very hard in the beginning to understand that the whole idea is not to beat the other runners. Eventually you learn that the competition is against the little voice inside you that wants to quit.

— GEORGE SHEEHAN

When I first started running, I was so embarrassed I'd walk when cars passed me. I'd pretend I was looking at the flowers.

— JOAN BENOIT SAMUELSON

Running is the classical road to self-consciousness, self-awareness, and self-reliance.

— NOEL CARROLL

———⋆◆⋆———

My first understanding was that you could not become a distance runner quickly. I began gradually, not doing too much.

— HENRY RONO

———⋆◆⋆———

I believe in gradual experimentation with running shoes.

— BILL RODGERS

———⋆◆⋆———

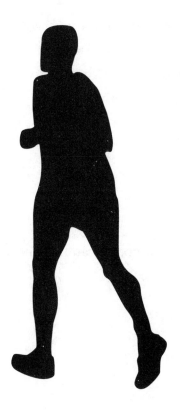

Running is the most elemental sport there is. We are genetically programmed to do it. One might even say we are the free-ranging, curious, restless creatures that we are because of running.

— JOHN JEROME, *THE ELEMENTS OF EFFORT*

Not just exercise, but a way to get in touch with and reclaim myself in an often fragmenting world, running also serves as a powerful antidote to clinical depression, a metaphor for the creative process, and, in its most profound moments, a spiritual practice.

— ALISON TOWNSEND

What I tell women is that anybody can become a runner if she really wants to.

— PRISCILLA WELCH

I was running since I was ten. Since grade one at school, people looked at me and thought, oh gosh, she can really run, she's a natural.

— CATHY FREEMAN

Running is like going to a spring: Each of us drinks our fill, and new runners come, pushing aside those in front.

— MICHAEL SANDROCK

Running is the kind of sport where, once it becomes part of your daily routine, there's very little attrition. That's what sets the running boom apart from other booms.

— FRANK SHORTER

Too many people have refused to begin running or have quickly dropped out of running programs because they "have no talent for it." Ridiculous. Talent has nothing to do with it. The only thing that matters is mental discipline.

— AMBY BURFOOT, *THE PRINCIPLES OF RUNNING*

No one will burn out doing aerobic running. It is too much anaerobic running, which the American scholastic athletic system tends to put young athletes through, that burns them out.

— ARTHUR LYDIARD

On my first day as a runner, I owned nine motorcycles, two cars, a camper, a garden tractor, a riding lawn mower, and a gas-powered weed whacker. I was never in danger of having to exert myself.

— JOHN BINGHAM, *THE COURAGE TO START*

To change into my baggy shorts and faded Berkeley tank top with the rainbow across the chest, pull my purple running shoes on, and just go, out the door and away, my body emptied of anything but movement through air and what that movement makes of me.

— ALISON TOWNSEND

I found myself starting over and needed an outlet, a way to channel the seething debris of rage left over from the divorce and my slowly deteriorating self-esteem and confidence. Running seemed to fit the bill. That, and a martial arts program.

— DONNA ISAACSON

I protested that I was weak and not fit to run, but the coach sent me for a physical examination and the doctor said that I was perfectly well. So I had to run, and when I got started I felt I wanted to win. But I only came in second. That was the way it started.

— EMIL ZATOPEK

The creative juices can really start flowing when runners are immersed in the wonderful feeling that accompanies the rhythm of running.

— FLORENCE GRIFFITH JOYNER AND JOHN HANC, *RUNNING FOR DUMMIES*

My greatest challenge when I first started running was overcoming the stares I would get. I began running in 1967, and no other women were out there. I ran around a track and it was so uncomfortable because the men would make comments and I didn't like how they would look at me. I overcame it by running without my contact lenses and pretending the guys weren't there.

— RENITA, RUNNER FROM SARASOTA, FLORIDA

Set a goal and a program for yourself, and everything else will follow. Guaranteed.

— AMBY BURFOOT, *THE PRINCIPLES OF RUNNING*

When you experience the run, you regress back to the mandrill on the savannah eluding the enclosing pride of lions that is planning to take your very existence away.

— SHAWN FOUND

For the novice runner, I'd say to give yourself at least two months of consistently running several times a week at a conversational pace before deciding whether you want to stick with it. Consistency is the most important aspect of training at this point.

— FRANK SHORTER

We were meant to run, and we do so naturally when left to our own devices.

— AMBY BURFOOT, *THE RUNNER'S GUIDE TO THE MEANING OF LIFE*

Physical fitness is not only one of the most important keys to a healthy body, it is the basis of dynamic and creative intellectual activity.

— JOHN F. KENNEDY

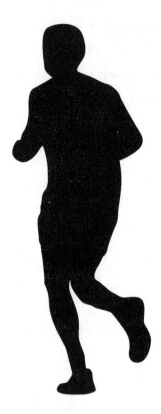

We're talking about a social movement. It was something that . . . was growing, the idea that you could train at any age, that almost anyone could run a marathon if they ran slow enough, and were patient and drank enough liquid along the way.

— KENNY MOORE ON THE BIRTH OF THE RUNNING MOVEMENT IN
  THE 1970S

It did not have a spokesman yet. It was still a private thing, where you snuck off to run in old sweats.

— KENNY MOORE

———⟫⬦⟪———

Fitness has to be fun. If it is not play, there will be no fitness. Play, you see, is the process. Fitness is merely the product.

— GEORGE SHEEHAN

———⟫⬦⟪———

[I]n running (like religion), it's the converts who are likely to exhibit the most zeal. And for that reason, the continuing influx of average beginning runners will always be the lifeblood of this sport.

— MARK WILL-WEBER

———⟫⬦⟪———

I run because I am an animal. I run because it is part of my genetic wiring. I run because millions of years of evolution have left me programmed to run. And, finally, I run because there's no better way to see the sun rise and set.

— AMBY BURFOOT, *THE RUNNER'S GUIDE TO THE MEANING OF LIFE*

Everyone who has run knows that its most important value is in removing tension and allowing a release from whatever other cares the day may bring.

— JIMMY CARTER

Why should I practice running slow? I already know how to run slow. I want to learn to run fast.

— EMIL ZATOPEK

I always tell beginning runners: Train your brain first. It's much more important than your heart or legs.

— AMBY BURFOOT, *THE PRINCIPLES OF RUNNING*

In short, running can change your entire outlook on life and make a new person out of you.

— MARC BLOOM, *THE RUNNER'S BIBLE*

When I got to the starting line, I didn't even know where to stand.

— GRETE WAITZ, *RUN YOUR FIRST MARATHON*

Non-runners may not believe how beneficial running can be, but it's true. Running has rocked people's lives—improving the way they look, the way they feel, the way they think, and the way they look at life.

> — FLORENCE GRIFFITH JOYNER AND JOHN HANC, *RUNNING FOR DUMMIES*

Look at me: a natural distance runner, wiry and muscular, trained down to gristle. We are the *infantry* of running. Your four-forty and eight-eighty men, these are your cavalry. The sprinters are your shock troops, your commandos.

> — JOHN L. PARKER, JR., *ONCE A RUNNER*

You don't need any skill to run. . . . Every 3-year-old knows how to run.

> — AMBY BURFOOT, *THE RUNNER'S GUIDE TO THE MEANING OF LIFE*

I always cringe inside when people say running comes naturally to me, that training is an uplifting joy. That's not why I race well. I'm competitive.

— EAMONN COGHLAN

—◆—

May your road ahead be a smooth one.

— GRETE WAITZ AND GLORIA AVERBUCH, *RUN YOUR FIRST MARATHON*

—◆—

The longer the stride the better, but one must never try to take long strides. To overstride oneself is the world of all faults in running, and it is certain to happen if the runner attempts to lengthen his stride.

— HARRY ANDREWS

—◆—

When running for exercise and not competition, you should run at an even pace that allows you to talk comfortably. If you run too fast and get breathless, you may not be able to go the distance.

— *THE U.S. NAVY SEAL GUIDE TO FITNESS AND NUTRITION*

There are no longer true amateurs in track.

— ADRIAN PAULEN, INTERNATIONAL AMATEUR ATHLETICS FOUNDATION PRESIDENT

Problems begin when expectations exceed ability.

— JONATHAN BEVERLY

I wasn't nervous the first time because I didn't know what to be nervous about. I had no idea what I was in for.

— GRETE WAITZ, *RUN YOUR FIRST MARATHON*

Running has taught me, perhaps more than anything else, that there's no reason to fear starting lines . . . or other new beginnings.

— AMBY BURFOOT, *THE RUNNER'S GUIDE TO THE MEANING OF LIFE*

If you have ever been around a runner who has just broken a barrier— say suddenly being able to run a 10-,9-,8-, or 7-minute mile—then you understand the magic.

— JEFF GALLOWAY

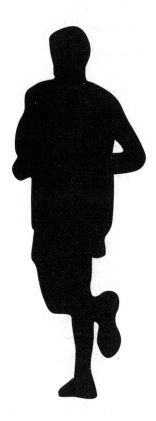

I could run very fast. After all, in Alabama, all we kids had to do was run, so we ran.

— JESSE OWENS

As the noted saying goes—training is 90 percent physical and 10 percent mental, but look out for that 10 percent.

— GRETE WAITZ AND GLORIA AVERBUCH, *RUN YOUR FIRST MARATHON*

———◆———

That's the beauty of starting lines: Until you begin a new venture, you never know what awaits you.

— AMBY BURFOOT, *THE RUNNER'S GUIDE TO THE MEANING OF LIFE*

———◆———

CHAPTER TWO

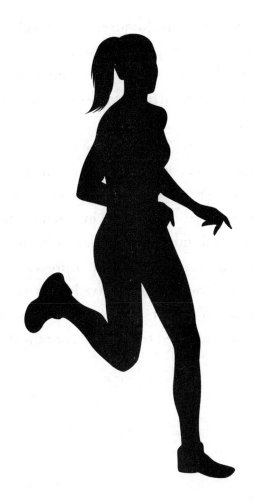

The running personality

Running to Form

The human body consists of one hundred trillion cells. That is a number so immense that the mind within that body almost cannot comprehend it. But when we lace our shoes, step through the door and move into the environment to engage in the activity we love most, every one of those cells shifts into motion.

They are put in motion by the heart. Not the heart of cardiologists, but the heart of philosophers, who look within the body and even within the mind. "The desire to run comes from deep within us," wrote Dr. Sheehan, "from the unconscious, the instinctive, the intuitive."

I became a runner for admittedly mundane reasons while a sophomore in high school: to win a letter in track and impress my girlfriend of the moment. The letter and the girlfriend have long passed from my life, but running remains a part of that life and always will as long as I have the heart to push those one hundred trillion cells out the door each day.

We are different, in essence, from other men.

— EMIL ZATOPEK

———◆◆———

Coffee doesn't do it for me; it's running that gets me going.

— JOAN BENOIT SAMUELSON

———◆◆———

I am very determined and the sport is my passion. I believe I am born for running.

— CATHY FREEMAN

———◆◆———

Running isn't simply a discipline. It can become like a compulsion—it can become like a god. If you worship this god, you forget everything else. And when you lose this god, you've got nothing.

— ALBERTO SALAZAR

———◆◆———

To run a world record, you have to have the absolute arrogance to think you can run a mile faster than anyone who's ever lived; and then you have to have the absolute humility to actually do it.

— HERB ELLIOTT

It takes a lot more than ability to run fast; it takes the ability to keep coming back and keep coming back.

— BENJI DURDEN

I run, therefore I am. And given the years improved fitness adds to our lives, if I did not run, maybe I would no longer be.

— HAL HIGDON

Even when I'm running I smile because I know that I don't have to.

— JOHN BINGHAM, "WHO NEEDS A REASON?" *RUNNERS WORLD*

———

"Women have more stamina," she said. "I knew it before liberation."

— NURSE PHILLIPS IN MAX APPLE'S "CARBO-LOADING"

———

I ran and ran every day, and I acquired a sense of determination, this sense of spirit that I would never, never, give up, no matter what else happened.

— WILMA RUDOLPH

———

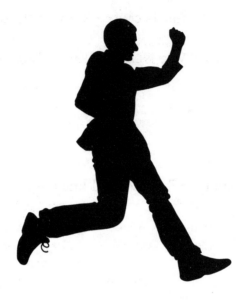

I am fanatical about my socks.

— KIM AHRENS

❖

Nothing gets in the way of my workout.

— ROBERT DE CASTELLA

❖

[Running] pervades my life. I wouldn't go so far as to say it has crept into other parts of my life; I would rather say it has become its own part of my life.

— LARRY SMITH

I've always got such high expectations for myself. I'm aware of them, but I can't relax them.

— MARY DECKER SLANEY

The desire to run comes from deep within us—from the unconscious, the instinctive, the intuitive.

— GEORGE SHEEHAN

Why did I get seriously involved in running? I can't put my finger on one specific thing. I became a runner because it suited my personality. It suited me as an individual. There may be a lot of different reasons, but, somehow, they all came together.

— BILL RODGERS

What am I doing—nobody cares. It's just personal satisfaction.

— KENNY MOORE, AMERICAN FOURTH-PLACE FINISHER IN THE 1972 OLYMPIC MARATHON

Every run is a great run!

— SASHA AZEVEDO

Like so many runners, if I don't run, I don't feel right. I don't feel relaxed; I don't enjoy eating.

— FRED LEBOW

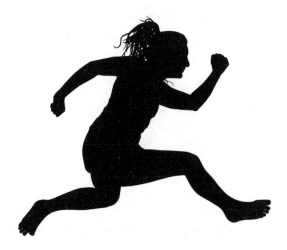

The key ingredient, in my opinion, to successful mental training is what I refer to as a "warrior attitude."

— BOB GLOVER AND SHELLY-LYNN FLORENCE GLOVER, *THE COMPETITIVE RUNNER'S HANDBOOK*

On those mornings when I was tempted to roll over and fall asleep again, I imagined my racing rivals leaping out of bed and roaring out the front door on a ten-mile workout. The thought so terrified me that I was generally lacing up my shoelaces within five minutes.

— AMBY BURFOOT

I began running after I became a writer. Since being a writer requires sitting at a desk for hours, I figured that without exercising I'd get out of shape. That was twenty-two years ago.

— HARUKI MURAKAMI

The thing I have always liked best about runners is the camaraderie.

— KATHRINE SWITZER

Running is such a part of my life. If I were never to run another marathon, I would still do two-hour runs.

— JOAN BENOIT SAMUELSON

It's common for runners to have failed at other sports. They're often slight, and sometimes not coordinated either.

— BENJAMIN CHEEVER, *STRIDES*

Passion is pushing myself when there is no one else around—just me and the road.

— RYAN SHAY

With the huge growth of our sport we don't have to train in solitude. Most runners will improve not just their fitness but also their enjoyment of running by teaming up with others.

— BOB GLOVER, *THE RUNNER'S HANDBOOK*

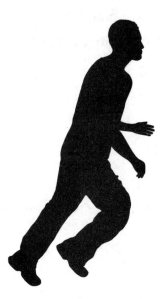

Eating is not a commitment, it is just something you do. That's what running is to me.

— LARRY SMITH

=—◆—=

[R]unning asks that I engage in a practice as difficult, disciplined, and liberating as the writing I do much of the rest of the time.

— ALISON TOWNSEND

=—◆—=

My upbringing gave me a strong will, a mental aggressiveness in what I wanted to achieve.

— PAUL TERGAT

They knew him only as another of those crazy runners who goes out every day to punish himself into a state of fitness. And to give the dogs and the motorists fits.

— BRUCE TUCKMAN, "LONG ROAD TO BOSTON"

No one can say, "You must not run faster than this, or jump higher than that." The human spirit is indomitable.

— ROGER BANNISTER

A guy who has run twenty Boston Marathons was once asked, "Don't you feel like skipping a day when it's raining?" The old road warrior replied, "If you start skipping runs because the weather's too lousy, pretty soon you start missing runs because the weather's too nice!"

— FLORENCE GRIFFITH JOYNER AND JOHN HANC, *RUNNING FOR DUMMIES*

Every day, I stop halfway through my run for five minutes, look around, and enjoy the surroundings. I'm reminded of why I do this and why I love it so much.

— ANITA ORTIZ

[W]hen you actually race [famous runners], you don't want to hear about their being the stuff of legend. You want flesh and blood, preferably flesh covered with a slothful six or seven percent body fat and blood running a little low on hemoglobin. You want to see an arm action start to labor, a back stiffen. You want mortality, not legend.

— KENNY MOORE

I didn't enjoy running at first. I thought it was boring. Running in soccer was part of the game so it was okay, but not running for the sake of running.

— RAY STEFFEN

There is nothing quite so gentle, deep, and irrational as our running— and nothing quite so savage, and so wild.

— BERND HEINRICH, *WHY WE RUN: A NATURAL HISTORY*

Non-runners can add some counterbalance to our fanaticism. Show me a real runner and I will show you someone who has, at least on occasion, become too wrapped up in the sport.

— MARK WILL-WEBER

I always run alone, away from phones and stress. Running is a major part of my life because it keeps me sane.

— MICHAEL ROUX, JR., EXECUTIVE CHEF, LE GAVROCHE, LONDON

People ask why I run. I say, "If you have to ask, you will never understand." It is something only those select few know. Those who put themselves through pain, but know, deep down, how good it really feels.

— ERIN LEONARD

No other sport is as democratic as running.

— FLORENCE GRIFFITH JOYNER AND JOHN HANC, *RUNNING FOR DUMMIES*

You talk to enough runners, you'll find out how superstitious many of us are.

— DICK BEARDSLEY

⸻

I think it's good to be able to drive yourself.

— PRISCILLA WELCH

⸻

Years ago, the picture of people running marathons was these lean, mean Type-A male running machines, but today people running are your neighbors, just regular people.

— TRACY SUNDLUN, EXECUTIVE VICE PRESIDENT, ELITE RACING

⸻

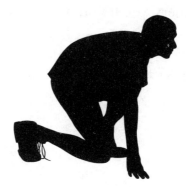

Colin saw that he was no racer but a runner, and a Narcissus among runners at that; he ran for the pleasure of watching himself move.

— VICTOR PRICE, "THE OTHER KINGDOM"

The training is my secret and if I told you what it was, it wouldn't be a secret anymore! I keep the secret in my heart.

— WILSON BOIT KIPKETER

Your toughness is made up of equal parts persistence and experience. You don't so much outrun your opponents as outlast and outsmart them, and the toughest opponent of all is the one inside your head.

— JOE HENDERSON

Coaching an elite runner is something like driving an expensive car. The coach's main job is to steer.

— JOHN BABINGTON

Runners are the Don Quixotes of the world, forever flailing at windmills, sometimes laughed at, rarely understood.

— MICHAEL SANDROCK

How would you describe the worst run you ever had? Precious!

— HAL HIGDON

You don't run against a bloody stopwatch. . . . A runner runs against himself, against the best that's in him. Not against a dead thing of wheels and pulleys. That's the way to be great, running against yourself. Against all the rotten mess in the world. Against God, if you're good enough.

— BILL PERSONS

In America, for example, sports have a "big bully" mentality. For instance, if you find a person who is good at running, he is usually small and wimpy. He runs away from other kids and is called a wimp. In Finland, we look at him as being an athlete who is good at running.

— EINO ROMPPANEN

A miler is the aristocrat of running. A miler is the closest thing to a thoroughbred horse that exists on two legs.

— JOHN L. PARKER, JR., *ONCE A RUNNER*

Running is the perfect sport for business travelers. While on location in Los Angeles, I actually bought one of those maps that show the celebrity homes and ran around looking for them.

— JILL CORDES

Running allows me to recharge my batteries. A good run adds a little bounce to my step.

— GEORGE W. BUSH

The records fell easily at first. Dozens of seconds peeled away with every running of a course, and I could hardly wait for the next chance to improve.

— JOE HENDERSON

The footing was really atrocious. I loved it.

— LYNN JENNINGS

"You, sir, are the greatest athlete in the world."
"Thanks, King."

— EXCHANGE BETWEEN GUSTAV V OF SWEDEN AND JIM THORPE AT THE 1912 OLYMPICS

Running fast is more fun than running slow.

— FRANK SHORTER

———◆———

Independence is the outstanding characteristic of the runner.

— NOEL CARROLL

———◆———

There is an itch in runners.

— ARNOLD HANO

———◆———

Why runners make lousy communists. In a word, individuality. It's the one characteristic all runners, as different as they are, seem to share. . . . Stick with it. Push yourself. Keep running. And you'll never lose that wonderful sense of individuality you now enjoy. Right, comrade?

— ADVERTISEMENT AT THE 1984 OLYMPICS

Learn to run when feeling the pain: then push harder.

— WILLIAM SIGEI

I was pushed by myself because I have my own rule, and that is that every day I run faster, and try harder.

— WILLIAM KIPKETER

I raced supremely well. I felt I was as well fitted to do it as I had ever been, and as perhaps I might ever be. I went climbing three weeks before, because I was feeling fed up with running.

— ROGER BANNISTER

Now some people like to act like things come easy to them, won't let on that they practice. Not me. I'll high-prance down 34th Street like a rodeo pony to keep my knees strong even if it does get my mother uptight so that she walks ahead like she's not with me, don't know me, is all by herself on a shopping trip and I am somebody else's crazy child.

— TONI CADE BAMBARA, "RAYMOND'S RUN"

When he did stop, to walk, it was like being a snail. Everything just . . . took . . . so . . . damn . . . looooonnngggg.

— RICHARD CHRISTIAN MATHESON, "THIRD WIND"

[H]e knows no fear and will not listen to the warnings we hopelessly recite: the jarred spine, ruined cartilage, wrecked knees and ankles, fractured shins, the mysterious sudden heart attack in the bloom of life, the neck broken on the expensive beach. . .

— LEN OTTO, "WE CANNOT SAVE HIM"

A coach can be like an oasis in the desert of a runner's lost enthusiasm.

— KEN DOHERTY

Coaching is an art and I'm not going to let anyone change me.

— MARTY STERN

Somehow, from plodding around in country track meets where 5:30 was dandy time for the one-mile run, the boy had wanted to be a runner. He had that craving for the feel of a level track and the thrill of a race— however he'd come by it, he had it.

— EDDY ORCUTT, "WHEELBARROW"

Except for .001 percent of the running population, everyone's in the same exact position: there will always be people slower than you, and people faster.

— "ASK MILES," *RUNNER'S WORLD*

The coach's main job is 20 percent technical and 80 percent inspirational.

— FRANZ STAMPFL

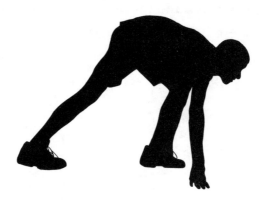

Is it raining? That doesn't matter. Am I tired? That doesn't matter, either. Then willpower will be no problem.

— EMIL ZATOPEK

A teacher is never too smart to learn from his pupils. But while runners differ, basic principles never change. So it's a matter of fitting your current practices to fit the event and the individual. See, what's good for you might not be worth a darn for the next guy.

— BILL BOWERMAN

As far as being a coach, it's always fascinated me. It's a greater responsibility than most people give it credit for because you're dealing with people.

— STEVE PREFONTAINE

I was always a great bundle of energy. As a child, instead of walking, I would run. And so running, which is a pain to a lot of people, was always a pleasure to me because it was so easy.

— ROGER BANNISTER

For me, running is a great way to jump-start my day, boost my energy, and have a few minutes to plan and prioritize my schedule.

— MICHAEL DELL

The greatest stimulator of my running career was fear.

— HERB ELLIOTT

———◆———

[The runner] must be a fanatic for hard work and enthusiastic enough to enjoy it.

— FRANZ STAMPFL

———◆———

I was a very driven kid, and I had much discipline, and I'd do anything to improve.

— GABE JENNINGS

———◆———

I'm not interested in athletics, I'm only interested in achievement.
Fix your goal and work for it.

— PERCY CERUTTY'S TRAINING ADVICE TO HERB ELLIOTT

We honor them all [famous runners] according to how well they honored
their own individuality.

— KENNY MOORE

My running was very simple: it was out of myself. Perhaps sometimes I
was like a mad dog. It didn't matter about style or what it looked like to
others; there were records to break.

— EMIL ZATOPEK

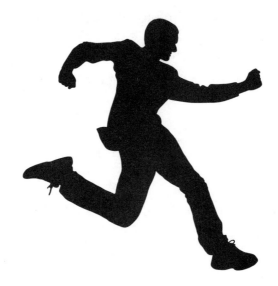

I have met my hero, and he is me.

— GEORGE SHEEHAN

———✦———

Since I'd read *Walden* in high school, I had been haunted by Thoreau's charge that when I came to die, I might discover that I had not lived. *If I ran a marathon*, I thought, *I will have lived.* I also thought I might die.

— BENJAMIN CHEEVER, *STRIDES*

———✦———

The true competitive runner, simmering in his own existential juices, endured his melancholia the only way he knew how; gently, together with those few others who also endured it, yet very much alone.

— JOHN L. PARKER, JR., *ONCE A RUNNER*

I love testing myself more than I fear being beaten, and front running is the ultimate test. You need total, irrevocable commitment to see the race through to the end or it cannot justify your effort.

— RON CLARKE

I like it, the way I live, but I can't explain the satisfaction to people who do not run. . . . Once you know international racing, you can't just ease off a bit. It has to be one or the other, as hard as you can, or just for fun.

— GRETE WAITZ

It may seem odd to hear a coach say this, but I think a really great training partner is more important than a coach.

— JOAN NESBIT, COACH AND WORLD-CLASS RUNNER

All my life people have been telling me, 'You're too small, Pre,' 'You're not fast enough, Pre,' 'Give up your foolish dream, Steve.' But they forget something: I have to win.

— STEVE PREFONTAINE

I've never known a runner who had as much patience as he needed.

— AMBY BURFOOT, *THE RUNNER'S GUIDE TO THE MEANING OF LIFE*

It's something in me, deep down, that makes me different in a race.

— EAMONN COGHLAN

———◆———

Any kind of athlete, dancer, gymnast, or figure skater is dependent on the body, not on a machine. It's very pure. You can't hide it.

— MICHELLE GIFFORD IN *NEW YORK CITY BALLET WORKOUT*

———◆———

Running is a way of life for me, just like brushing my teeth. If I don't run for a few days, I feel as if something's been stolen from me.

— JOHN A. KELLEY

———◆———

We're all professionals. Rules don't mean anything.

— FRANK SHORTER, TESTIFYING BEFORE THE PRESIDENT'S COMMISSION ON OLYMPIC SPORTS

———◆———

I was born to run. I love to run. It's almost like the faster I go, the easier it becomes.

— MARY DECKER SLANEY

———◆———

CHAPTER THREE

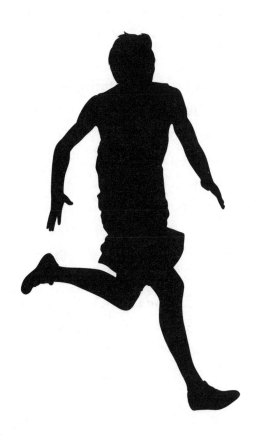

Tips, advice, and other observations

Going Into Training

What is the difference between running and training? Many runners probably do not even realize that there might be a difference, but one does exist. Running is simply when you run. Training is when you run with a purpose, a goal, a target at the end of the tunnel, be it a 5-K race or a marathon.

We often attach ourselves to both definitions. We run. We train. Some days we cross-train. And some days we rest, which is a form of training in the sense that you occasionally must rest your muscles so that you may run or train or cross-train again. We might do one or the other on any given day, or week, or year, or career.

Perhaps this makes running more complicated that it need be. Fortunately for those who prefer to strain their muscles rather than strain their brains, a wide body of literature exists telling them how to run or train or cross-train and when to rest. Books. Magazine articles. Training programs on the Internet that you can download into your computer or print and post on your refrigerator to guide you on your daily journeys.

All praise those who guide us.

Everyone is an athlete. The only difference is that some of us are in training, and some are not.

— GEORGE SHEEHAN

Training is principally an act of faith. The athlete must believe in its efficacy: he must believe that through training he will become fitter and stronger.

— FRANZ STAMPFL

What I did in those early months wasn't "training." It was more about trying not to get hurt than trying to get better.

— JOHN BINGHAM, *NO NEED FOR SPEED: A BEGINNER'S GUIDE TO THE JOY OF RUNNING*

Running is one of the best solutions to a clear mind.

— SASHA AZEVEDO

⟞⟐⟝

Training of female athletes is so new that the limits of female possibility are still unknown.

— KATHERINE DUNN

⟞⟐⟝

What the years have shown me is that running clarifies the thinking process as well as purifies the body. I think best—most broadly and fully—when I am running.

— AMBY BURFOOT, *THE RUNNER'S GUIDE TO THE MEANING OF LIFE*

⟞⟐⟝

Two months before the 1952 Olympic Games in Helsinki, the doctors said I must not compete. I had a gland infection in my neck. Well, I didn't listen and what happened? Three golds.

— EMIL ZATOPEK

Putting miles in your training log is like putting money in the bank. You begin to draw interest on it immediately.

— HAL HIGDON

Injuries made me a cross-training believer.

— FLORENCE GRIFFITH JOYNER

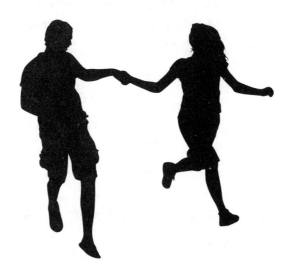

In place of wasteful hobbies there commences a period of supervised and systematic physical training, together with instruction in the art of living fully. This replaces previously undirected life.

— ONE OF PERCY CERUTTY'S TRAINING RULES

If you can train your mind for running, everything else will be easy.

— AMBY BURFOOT

In my opinion, nothing beats a treadmill workout when you don't want to run outside. A good movie, some water, and a little ventilation are all you need.

— FLORENCE GRIFFITH JOYNER

To exercise at or near capacity is the best way I know of reaching a true introspective state. If you do it right, it can open all kinds of inner doors.

— AL OERTER

At the highest level, it's interesting to think of what, out of all the training, makes the difference. In Joanie's case, it was running those certain loops very fast.

— FRANK SHORTER ON JOAN BENOIT SAMUELSON

As time goes on, I am more into alternative training.

— GRETE WAITZ

———◆———

[M]ost of my early training was experimental. I tested theories and techniques on myself. If they worked, I'd pass them on to my friends.

— TED CORBITT

———◆———

Of course, I know all the gear in the world won't make me a better runner. Only time and effort do that. But all the gadgets over the years have sure made my training a lot more interesting—and fun.

— JOHN BINGHAM, "READY FOR TAKEOFF," *RUNNERS WORLD*

———◆———

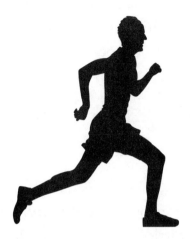

To familiarize themselves with pain, slaves flogged their backs with rhododendron branches until they bled.

— THE TRAINING PRACTICE OF ANCIENT ROMAN ATHLETES

Not all training is good or desirable; very much is unquestionably injurious.

— *LONDON SOCIETY* IN 1864

First, I figured out the time I thought the mile should be run in. Second, I started testing my theories and particularly my own constitution and capabilities; the result of this study soon convinced me that the then existing records at the distance were by no means good.

— WALTER GEORGE

We are obviously not far from our limit of safety. If we doubled our speed of movement . . . athletics would become a highly dangerous pastime.

— ARCHIBALD HILL IN 1927 ON THE DANGERS OF TOO MUCH RUNNING

The most important day in any running program is rest. Rest days give your muscles time to recover so you can run again. Your muscles build in strength as you rest.

— HAL HIGDON

Two- and three-mile events are my objective at the moment. I am out to build up stamina and only racing in those events will help me. It was stamina that beat me when I was away at the Games, and I do not want it to happen again.

— JOHN LANDY

By changing the training techniques and attitudes that had previously dominated running, [Bill Bowerman, Kenneth Cooper, and Arthur Lydiard] helped make it possible for running to be more than a sport for elite young athletes (nearly all of them male).

— JOE HENDERSON, *RUNNING 101*

[Running] transported him, taking his mind to another place, very deep within. Like prayer.

— RICHARD CHRISTIAN MATHESON, "THIRD WIND"

[Scientific testing] can't determine how the mind will tolerate pain in a race. Sometimes, I say, "Today I can die."

— GELINDO BORDIN

The essential thing in life is not so much conquering as fighting well.

— BARON DE COUBERTIN, FOUNDER OF THE MODERN OLYMPIC GAMES

The ability to concentrate is the single element that separates the merely good athlete from the great ones. Concentration is the hallmark of the elite runner.

— WILLIAM P. MORGAN

Training is like putting money in a bank. You deposit money, and then you can take it out.

— FRED LEBOW

It's like a car starting. There's an immense amount of energy you need to start the car, but once you're rolling, it's easy.

— JOHN LANDY ON STARTING TRAINING

The battles that count aren't the ones for gold medals. The struggles within yourself—the invisible, inevitable battles inside all of us—that's where it's at.

— JESSE OWENS

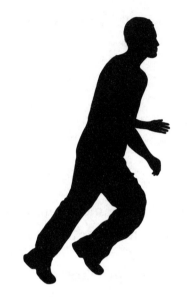

The human body can do so much. Then the heart and spirit must take over.

— Sohn Kee-Chung, winner of the 1936 Olympic Marathon

When running to fill a time quota . . . you can't make that time pass any faster by rushing, so you settle into a pace that feels right to you at the moment. Each minute above a quota is a little victory.

— JOE HENDERSON

If you talk to an elite or near-elite American distance runner today, they'll tell you that the primary aim of their training is to avoid injury. If you had talked to a similar athlete 25 years ago—somebody doing the '82 Boston, for example—he would have told you the idea of training was to run fast.

— TOM DERDERIAN, COACH OF THE GREATER BOSTON TRACK CLUB

A lot of people think that they can "sweat out" a fever by running. They think that running will help their immune system fight it off. That's wrong.

— DAVID NIEMAN, PH.D., HEAD OF THE HUMAN PERFORMANCE LABORATORY, APPALACHIAN STATE UNIVERSITY

Everyone who competes goes into strict training. They do it to get a crown that will not last; but we do it to get a crown that will last forever. Therefore, I do not run like a man running aimlessly.

— ST. PAUL IN HIS LETTER TO THE CORINTHIANS 9:24

There are as many ways to be successful as a distance runner as there are athletes. You have to develop a training schedule of your own.

— CRAIG VIRGIN

The thinking must be done first, before training begins.

— PETER COE

He entertained the fervent wish that a bolt of lightning would shoot from the sky and strike him dead on the spot, ending his pain. But another part of him wished for the strength to accelerate, to take off like he did at the start of his morning runs, fresh and energetic after a night's sleep.

— BRUCE TUCKMAN, "LONG ROAD TO BOSTON"

Training is different from just plain running. It's the difference between tossing the football around every other day and trying out for the team.

— MARC BLOOM, *THE RUNNER'S BIBLE*

Say no to "no pain, no gain" and instead "train, don't strain."

— BOB GLOVER, *THE RUNNER'S HANDBOOK*

Long slow distance makes long slow runners.

— Jim Bush, coach at UCLA

Hills are speedwork in disguise.

— Frank Shorter

Running is "focusing" for me. In my profession we might talk about it as body prayer; a sort of emptying of the mind. That's probably why I prefer running in the wilds rather than in the city.

— Most Reverend Katherine Jefferts Schori, Presiding Bishop, the Episcopal Church, New York City

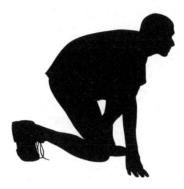

With the proper motivation, that is, a good reason for wanting to do it, your mind can overcome any sort of adversity.

— FRANZ STAMPFL

Don't judge your running by your speed.

— AMBY BURFOOT, *THE PRINCIPLES OF RUNNING*

Hill training is often more of a mental challenge than a physical one.

— FLORENCE GRIFFITH JOYNER

Strange how he never got hungry on these marathons of his. The body just seemed to live off itself for the period of time it took. Next day he usually put away a supermarket, but in running, all appetite faded. The body fed itself.

— RICHARD CHRISTIAN MATHESON, "THIRD WIND"

You don't need a $100 pair of shoes. It's not running that's damaging to the body, it's running badly. And shoes just encourage that.

— KEN BOB SAXTON, FOUNDER OF RUNNINGBAREFOOT.ORG, WHO HAS COMPLETED ABOUT 35 MARATHONS AND ULTRAS WITHOUT SHOES

Maybe wearing heavy boots in training and light shoes in competition was good; when you change, whoosh. It was very practical.

— EMIL ZATOPEK ON WEARING CZECH ARMY-ISSUE MILITARY BOOTS IN TRAINING

He trained to do it differently. And people couldn't respond. However he got in a position to do that, he did. What happens is the change in the psychological process in the race.

— FRANK SHORTER ON HOW LASSE VIREN CHANGED RACING TACTICS

There is no substitute for learning to live in our bodies. All the tests and all the machines in the world will fail if we do not first become good animals.

— GEORGE SHEEHAN

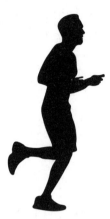

When I am training and competing, I really concentrate, but during the rest of the day, I don't want to think about running.

— INGRID KRISTIANSEN

Every runner has a perfect training level of weekly miles that will allow him or her to maximize performance and minimize injuries. Finding that level is not always easy to do.

— HAL HIGDON

Dancing and running shake up the chemistry of happiness.

— MASON COOLEY

———◆———

Everything changed the day I understood that if I was to become a runner, I would have to run with the body I had.

— JOHN BINGHAM, *THE COURAGE TO START*

———◆———

It's as if you set your destination [.. .] and then you figure out how you're getting there from where you are. So you plan your training and your diet, and figure out what else you need to do to get you from this point to that point.

— LORRAINE MOLLER

———◆———

The mind's first step to self-awareness must be made through the body.

— GEORGE SHEEHAN

Nonrunners cannot see how they can afford the time to run every day. But runners cannot imagine getting through a single day without it.

— KEVIN NELSON, *THE RUNNER'S BOOK OF DAILY INSPIRATION*

Everything I see and feel is more extreme when I'm in training. If I'm happy, I'm happier. If I'm sad, I'm sadder.

— KATHRINE SWITZER

I didn't get a chance to voice my opinion on whether or not I *wanted* to run. I'd joined the Women's Army Corps and when Aunt Sam yelled, "Double-time, march!" that's exactly what we all did—no matter if our feet were blistered and our lungs felt ready to pop.

— ROBERTA B. JACOBSON

It is amazing how much you can progress week after week, month after month, year after year if you allow for gradual training increases.

— BOB GLOVER, *THE RUNNER'S HANDBOOK*

If you under-train, you may not finish, but if you over-train, you may not start.

— STAN JENSEN

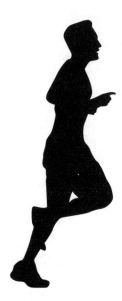

When I was a customer service representative for a bank the year before the 1988 Olympics, I had to make time to run: before I went to work, on my lunch hour, and after work. It was no easy task, but the results were great.

— FLORENCE GRIFFITH JOYNER

The more I train, the more I realize I have more speed in me.

— LEROY BURRELL

I looked at Paavo Nurmi and the rest of the great Finnish runners before the war, and I realized that what set them up, apart from the others of the day, was that they did high mileage.

— ARTHUR LYDIARD

Run like hell and get the agony over with.

— CLARENCE DeMAR

When you first get a hill in sight, look at the top of it only once. Then imagine yourself at the bottom of the other side.

— FLORENCE GRIFFITH JOYNER

Running was supposed to collapse my uterus.

— KATHRINE SWITZER ON AN OLD WIVES' TALES ABOUT WHY SHE
    SHOULDN'T RUN

Once upon a time, about twenty years ago to be precise, runners believed they didn't have to do anything but run.

— AMBY BURFOOT, *THE PRINCIPLES OF RUNNING*

What I was doing in the past was running my easy days too fast and not letting the body rest a bit, and then getting on the track and not putting in the times and the effort. And I was not fresh enough to enjoy what I was doing.

— PRISCILLA WELCH

He loved the ache that shrouded his torso and he even waited for the moment, a few minutes into the run, when a dull voltage would climb his body to his brain like a vine, reviving him.

— RICHARD CHRISTIAN MATHESON, "THIRD WIND"

You get very tired, and there was a certain amount of pain and you slow up. Your legs are so tired that you are in fact slowing. If you don't keep running, keep your blood circulating, the muscles stop pumping the blood back and you get dizzy.

— ROGER BANNISTER

We forget our bodies to the benefit of mechanical leisure. We act continuously with our brain, but we no longer use our bodies, our limbs.

— EMIL ZATOPEK

Fitness is like the blade of a knife; you want to sharpen it without ruining the blade.

— SALLY JENKINS, THE *WASHINGTON POST*

———◆———

Coming from a farming background, I saw nothing out of the ordinary in running barefoot, although it seemed to startle the rest of the athletics world. I have always enjoyed going barefoot and when I was growing up I seldom wore shoes, even when I went into town.

— ZOLA BUDD

———◆———

For me, a seven-minute-a-mile pace is fast enough, and I often run slower. I'll sometimes start a workout running an eight-minute or nine-minute pace. You can achieve a lot with slow workouts.

— DOUG KURTIS

———◆———

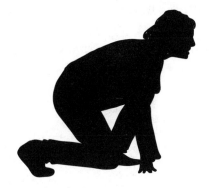

The worst injury I ever had was a stress fracture from running.

— GRETE WAITZ

———◆———

Run too far and the body doesn't want to stop.

— RICHARD CHRISTIAN MATHESON, "THIRD WIND"

———◆———

My training was very simple and very primitive.

— EMIL ZATOPEK ON HIS EARLY TRAINING

Spirit has fifty times the strength and staying power of brawn and muscle.

— ANONYMOUS

Once you're beat mentally, you might as well not even go to the starting line.

— TODD WILLIAMS, TOP AMERICAN DISTANCE RUNNER

In running it is man against himself, the cruelest of opponents. The other runners are not the real enemies. His adversary lies within him, in his ability with brain and heart to master himself and his emotions.

— GLENN CUNNINGHAM, AMERICAN RUNNER IN THE 1930s. HE WAS
SEVERELY BURNED IN CHILDHOOD AND ALMOST LOST HIS LEGS.

Racing teaches us to challenge ourselves. It teaches us to push beyond where we thought we could go. It helps us find out what we are made of.

— PATTI SUE PLUMER, AMERICAN OLYMPIAN IN THE 1992 OLYMPICS

We all have dreams. But in order to make dreams come into reality, it takes an awful lot of determination, dedication, self-discipline, and effort.

— JESSE OWENS

I have a resistance toward running.

— CHRISTY TURLINGTON

If I can get better, why not?

— EMIL ZATOPEK

When you're young and training two or three times a day, you can beat everybody your age, but you'll only last a few years.

— ARTURO BARRIOS

[The athlete] must believe that through training his perfomance will improve and continue to improve indefinitely for as long as he continues to train to progressively stiff standards.

— FRANZ STAMPFL

Mental toughness can take you to the top, and mental weakness straight to the bottom.

— JOHN SCHIEFER

⟨⟨━◆━⟩⟩

Every so often, if you find your times slowing down, if you find your strength leaving you a little bit, don't try to push through it. Totally detrain.

— PRISCILLA WELCH

⟨⟨━◆━⟩⟩

Leave your watch on the kitchen table and go—freely, like a child.

— CLAIRE KOWALCHIK, *THE COMPLETE BOOK OF RUNNING FOR WOMEN*

⟨⟨━◆━⟩⟩

You train best where you are the happiest.

— FRANK SHORTER

———◆———

I don't train. I just run my 3 to 15 miles a day.

— JACK FOSTER

———◆———

Races always evoke some dread about pain that will come. But we can't escape the fact that the more discomfort we accept in a race, the faster we will run. Successful racing means *courting the pain*.

— JOHN ELLIOTT

———◆———

My basic philosophy can be summed up by an expression we use in Norwegian: hurry slowly. Get there, but be patient.

— GRETE WAITZ, *RUN YOUR FIRST MARATHON*

———◆———

Never really give in as long as you have an earthly chance.

— ALF SHRUBB

———◆———

If the ancient men ran, then so did ancient women. Atalanta was left to die in the forest by a cruel father who had wanted a son. The babe was suckled by a bear. A hunter saw her racing through the wilderness and was astonished by her beauty and speed.

— BENJAMIN CHEEVER, *STRIDES*

———◆———

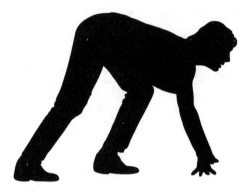

Many statistics say we only use a small percentage of our brains. I think the same can be said about the body.

— PETER MARTINS AND NEW YORK CITY BALLET, *NEW YORK CITY BALLET WORKOUT*

I learned, one, you shouldn't ever quit. And I learned, two, you'll never be able to explain it to anybody.

— JIM RYUN

Most people never run far enough on their first wind to find out they've got a second. Give your dreams all you've got and you'll be amazed at the energy that comes out of you.

— WILLIAM JAMES

When we run, we are already so exposed, often nearly naked in our shorts and T-shirts, huffing and puffing, purified by the effort. Briefly removed from the defenses and secrets we maintain in so much of our lives, we feel less need to hide our private thoughts, loves, fears, and stresses. We share.

— AMBY BURFOOT, *THE RUNNER'S GUIDE TO THE MEANING OF LIFE*

Never attempt to pass a man on a bend, always improve your position on the straight.

— HARRY ANDREWS

The man who can drive himself further once the effort gets painful is the man who will win.

— ROGER BANNISTER

You need great humility to run a marathon!

— GRETE WAITZ AND GLORIA AVERBUCH, *RUN YOUR FIRST MARATHON*

Success is the result of the application of scientific methods of training to the development of natural talents or skill, which we all possess in some degree or another.

— WALTER GEORGE

I never had technique.

— AL OERTER

———◆———

Running on an artificial leg at full speed is like driving backward at 55 miles per hour, using only your rearview mirror to guide you.

— THOMAS BOURGEOIS

———◆———

We train through the winter in deep snow and ice. Our slogan is "Pain is good, more pain is even better."

— MATT CARPENTER, MOUNTAIN RUNNER

———◆———

Pain, like time, is a backdrop to running.

— SALLY PONT

Accept the ups and downs you will experience. You are going to have days you feel like you're flying and days you struggle. This is normal for all runners.

— GRETE WAITZ AND GLORIA AVERBUCH, *RUN YOUR FIRST MARATHON*

I see elegance and beauty in every female athlete. I don't think being an athlete is unfeminine. I think of it as a kind of grace.

— JACKIE JOYNER-KERSEY

I have heard a million people say that running is the most boring activity that they can possibly imagine. Since I'm sure I'm not any smarter or wittier than these people, I can only guess that they never learned to listen as they run. If they did, they would surely be entertained and informed by their own thoughts.

— AMBY BURFOOT, *THE RUNNER'S GUIDE TO THE MEANING OF LIFE*

People train much harder than they did before . . . Is there a limit? Athletes don't think that way.

— BILL ROGERS

It is an aspect of training, but a subtle aspect. I don't think about it much.

— JIM RYUN, ON PAIN.

Now, how would you define a track athlete who spends all of his or her time training and competing, is paid to appear in meets, paid bonuses for good performances, paid to wear certain shoes, paid to say good things about corporate sponsors? Unless you are totally naïve and incredibly ignorant, or unless you have reason to twist the truth, "professional" would have to be your answer.

— CARL LEWIS

———⊰◆⊱———

Set aside a time solely for running. Running is more fun if you don't have to rush though it.

— JIM FIXX

———⊰◆⊱———

Track and field is not ice-skating. It is not necessary to smile and make a wonderful impression on the judges.

— EMIL ZATOPEK

———⊰◆⊱———

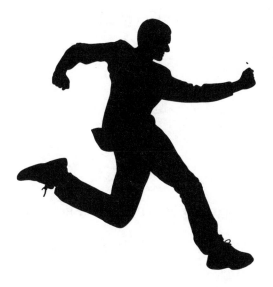
I got caught in Seoul, lost my gold medal, and I'm here to tell people in this country it's wrong to cheat, not to take it, and it's bad for your health. I started taking steroids when I was nineteen years old because most of the world-class athletes were taking drugs.

— BEN JOHNSON, WHO WAS STRIPPED OF AN OLYMPIC GOLD MEDAL FOR TESTING POSITIVE FOR STEROID USE.

I have a good time. I let my mind go blank.

— JIM RYUN

———◆———

I've learned that it's what you do with your miles, rather than how many you've run.

— ROD DeHAVEN

———◆———

CHAPTER FOUR

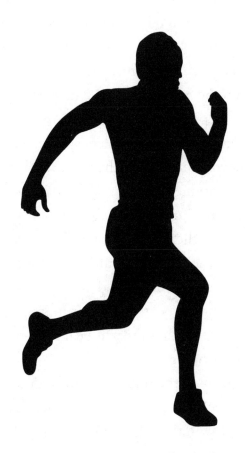

Our "Gigantic" running miscellany

Running with the Pack, Part I

Growing up as competitive athletes, we become inspired by great athletes who preceded us in the sport. The champion who inspired me most was one of the greatest, though his numerous world records long have been broken: Emil Zatopek of Czechoslovakia. Times aside, nobody has matched Zatopek's achievements, particularly at the 1952 Olympic Games when he won the 5,000 and 10,000 meters and the marathon.

As a middling runner at a small school in Minnesota (Carleton College), I read of the great Czech athlete's victories in *Track & Field News* and knew I never could attain the same level of glory.

Three years later, stationed with the U.S. Army in Germany, I attended a track meet in Furth featuring as its star performer Emil Zatopek, my hero. I was then not fast enough to receive an invitation to compete, so I hung on the fence surrounding the track to get as close as possible to the Czech as he effortlessly defeated a German opponent.

Each running step for the next year was run in pursuit of Emil Zatopek, not in expectation that I might beat him, but that I might narrow the time gap between us.

As chance would have it, the following summer I ran a 5,000 in Finland won by Zatopek the previous year. Much faster because of a year's hard training, I won though in inferior time. I had not defeated Emil Zatopek, but I was part of the chase pack.

Every one of the exceptional athletes quoted and mentioned in this chapter had a hero that propelled him or her in their training. We all run in the footsteps of those who were great before our time

An object at rest tends to stay at rest and an object in motion tends to stay in motion. . .

— NEWTON'S FIRST LAW OF MOTION

———⊰•⊱———

Whatever the pace, run softly, run tall.

— JOE HENDERSON, *RUNNING 101*

———⊰•⊱———

I was not very talented. My basic speed was low. Only with willpower was I able to reach this world-best standard in long-distance running.

— EMIL ZATOPEK

———⊰•⊱———

I run because I enjoy running. . . . There is nothing special about me.

— Hezekiah Kipchoge "Kip" Keino

———◆———

The further I got into training for health and fitness, which it was in the beginning, the better it got.

— Priscilla Welch

———◆———

I became a runner because it suited my personality. It suited me as an individual.

— Bill Rodgers

———◆———

With victory in hand, running at maximum effort becomes very difficult.

— FRANK SHORTER

—◆—

I just had to get to the line first. My coach said, "Get to the front with 600 meters left, and stay there." I did.

— LASSE VIREN

—◆—

The medal is not for yourself. It couldn't be done without the support and help of my people, runners, and coaches.

— ALBERTO JUANTORENA

—◆—

Whatever moves the other runners made, I knew I could respond.

— GRETE WAITZ

———

You're only a hamstring injury away from oblivion.

— STEVE JONES

———

When I was growing up I wasn't inspired to be a marathoner. It wasn't even in a little girl's vocabulary.

— LORRAINE MOLLER

———

I was now running for the tape, the mental agony of knowing I had hit my limit, of not knowing what was happening behind me. I was not to know they were fading, too.

— SEBASTIAN COE

———

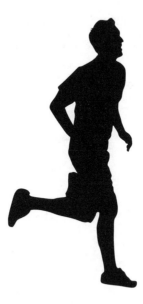

My goal was to figure out how I could win the Olympics. I had a plan and I trained with that goal in mind.

— LORRAINE MOLLER

This is what really matters: running. This is where I know where I am.

— STEVE JONES

When I am training and competing, I really concentrate, but during the rest of the day, I don't want to think about running.

— INGRID KRISTIANSEN

———◆———

Without some company in the difficult miles, the body's mission becomes lonely and dark.

— FRANK SHORTER

———◆———

I noted in my diary four or five things I did wrong in preparation for the race: like needing more 25-30 mile training runs, doing more speedwork, and drinking more fluids during a race. Unfortunately, I forgot all that at the Olympics.

— BILL RODGERS ON THE 1976 MONTREAL OLYMPICS

———◆———

The marathon is my only girlfriend. I give her everything I have.

— TOSHIHIKO SEKO

———◆———

The only secret is that it is consistent, often monotonous, boring, hard work. And it's tiring.

— ROBERT DE CASTELLA

———◆———

It changed my life enormously. I had my head so firmly planted in the sand. Now I see how flimsy life is.

— PRISCILLA WELCH ON HER CANCER DIAGNOSIS

———◆———

Intercollegiate track meets were not very important. . . . He used them as speed work. . . . He used them as stepping stones to the marathon.

— BILL RODGERS ON AMBY BURFOOT

I keep on running figuratively and literally, despite a limp that gets more noticeable with each passing season, because for me there has always been a place to go and a terrible urgency to get there.

— JOAN BENOIT SAMUELSON

I do everything I can to win.

— SAID AOUITA

I was motivated to win [the Boston Marathon] not only for myself, but for the Portuguese people of Boston. They were with me all the way and made winning this race the nicest moment of my life.

— ROSA MOTA

I train for good luck.

— ARTURO BARRIOS

I have the mentality that I can train like a man, and it helps me a lot.

— UTA PIPPIG

To really prove yourself in athletics nowadays, you have to stay 10 to 15 years. That's what I intend to do.

— NOUREDDINE MORCELI

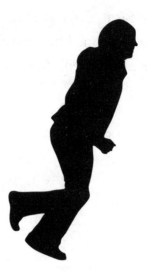

The little boy would take on boys twice his size and more often than not beat them in races round the school playground.

— FRANCIS NORONHA ON HEZEKIAH KIPCHOGE "KIP" KEINO

———⬦———

I simply decided to give running a go.

— PRISCILLA WELCH

———⬦———

Priscilla had a typical English childhood. She was no different than any of the other children in the area, though she was always full of energy as a child.

— BROTHER OF PRISCILLA WELCH

———

I liked running; it suited me physically and physiologically.

— BILL RODGERS

———

He was Thoreauvian, an organic gardener, a fan of Jack Kerouac.

— AMBY BURFOOT ON JOHN KELLEY

———

Like a kid on a playground, a wild-eyed look of wonder.

— BRUCE GOMEZ ON HOW BILL RODGERS LOOKED WHILE HE WAS RUNNING

———

People who make mistakes in the early miles by going out too hard or by not taking enough water are the ones who aren't going to win the race, or, perhaps, even finish it.

— BILL RODGERS

[O]f all the challenges I have faced, the greatest one has been the quest for combining my family and career.

— JOAN BENOIT SAMUELSON

He taught us that the essence of running was picking apples, jumping in water, and that kind of stuff.

— AMBY BURFOOT ON JOHN KELLEY

You can't rationalize performance.

— FRANK SHORTER

———⊰◆⊱———

Even though I may have been a bit of a layabout and smoked and drank or whatever, I always worked for my money.

— STEVE JONES

———⊰◆⊱———

He wasn't expected to do well, and always ran like he had something to prove.

— CLIVE THOMAS ON STEVE JONES

———⊰◆⊱———

I deliberately kept a low profile, because then I could quietly go about my business and do what I knew how to do best.

— LORRAINE MOLLER

———⊰◆⊱———

He didn't have the marathon bug. He didn't have the focus he developed later.

— AMBY BURFOOT ON BILL RODGERS IN COLLEGE

My career coincided with the evolution of women's distance running. I was able to get on at the beginning of it and ride it right through.

— LORRAINE MOLLER ON HER EARLY RUNNING CAREER

He was the first to transform the 5,000 and 10,000 into a protracted sprint. That is how he felt he was his best. Because before Lasse, nobody ever went that early.

— FRANK SHORTER ON HOW LASSE VIREN CHANGED RACING TACTICS

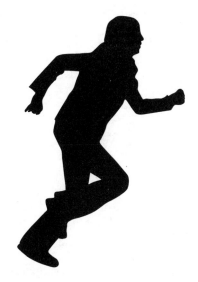

I never walked anywhere, it seems. I had a genuine, instinctive love of running.

— SEBASTIAN COE

—◆—

An athlete to a great extent determines his own training by his response to the tasks you set for him and by his racing results. The coach must adjust to his athlete.

— PETER COE ON TRAINING HIS SON, SEBASTIAN COE

—◆—

If you run too many races, you can run well, but not so many great races. And I like to do some real good races.

— INGRID KRISTIANSEN

———⊰•⊱———

When it was over, I told Scott, "Never again." But then again, I said the same thing after my first marathon.

— JOAN BENOIT SAMUELSON ON GIVING BIRTH TO HER DAUGHTER

———⊰•⊱———

Billy, slow down! Are you nuts?

— CHARLIE RODGERS TO BILL RODGERS AT THE 1975 BOSTON MARATHON

———⊰•⊱———

After that win I vowed never to question him again. I wasn't aware of what kind of shape he was in at the time.

> — CHARLIE RODGERS AFTER BILL RODGERS WON THE 1975 BOSTON MARATHON IN 2:09.55.

———

After my third place in Seoul, I want to prove I am the best. I will start indoors and then go outdoors.

> — SAID AOUITA

———

I don't know if it is paradise, but I think for someone like Said, it is very nice to go where he is respected, but where he can also live a reasonably normal life.

> — FRANK SHORTER ON SAID AOUITA IN BOULDER, COLORADO

———

In Mexico, when I was a kid, I never got exposed to different sports, like basketball, baseball, or tennis. In Mexico, it's not like it is in the United States, where you have the chance to play different sports. I'm happy with my choice, of course.

— ARTURO BARRIOS

It was a nice time, because I grew up not too serious in track and field. It was for fun.

— UTA PIPPIG ON HER CHILDHOOD

What about this silver?

— UTA PIPPIG'S FATHER WHEN SHE SHOWED HIM THE TEN GOLD AND ONE SILVER MEDAL SHE WON AT A TOWN SPORTS DAY AS A CHILD

I became a victim of the Norwegian expression "a silver medal is a defeat"—if you don't win, you lose.

— GRETE WAITZ

———◆———

Joan would have the feeling before the race that she wasn't afraid of anyone. Her way was to prepare so well.

— FRANK SHORTER ON JOAN BENOIT SAMUELSON

———◆———

I was in my last year in this apprentice home, and a race sponsored by the factory was organized across the city. I was obligated to take part. I wanted not to run.

— EMIL ZATOPEK ON HIS FIRST RACE, WHICH WAS SPONSORED BY THE SHOE FACTORY WHERE HE WAS AN APPRENTICE

———◆———

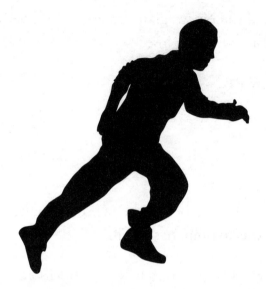

You can be compulsive until your first big orthopedic injury. Once you have that, you begin to think more.

— FRANK SHORTER

Like so many women, sometimes my needs and interests are congruous, and sometimes they compete with each other for my time, energy, and focus.

— JOAN BENOIT SAMUELSON

He ran with his head cocked to the side, as if he were listening to the others' footsteps, trying to determine if they were feeling as good as he was.

— MICHAEL SANDROCK ON STEVE JONES IN *RUNNING WITH THE LEGENDS*

———⊰◆⊱———

Just before 16 miles, de Castella looked across at me and surged. Every time he surged, I surged with him, and covered.

— STEVE JONES ON RUNNING AGAINST ROBERT DE CASTELLA

———⊰◆⊱———

It's much more difficult staying on top than getting there.

— ROBERT DE CASTELLA

———⊰◆⊱———

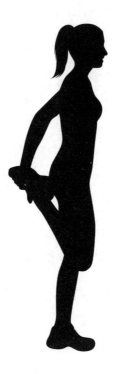

I realized he had talent. We'd go out on runs, and I had to work hard, concentrate on every stride; Bill would float along, with that vacant look in his eyes.

— AMBY BURFOOT ON BILL RODGERS AT WESLEYAN

Carlos was the best in the world, but he was not always at his best. He wasn't always consistent.

— STEVE JONES ON CARLOS LOPES

⬤

When I was a little girl, my parents said studying was the most important thing. "You need your job in the future, not sport," they told me. They couldn't believe running would be such a big thing for me.

— UTA PIPPIG

⬤

When you feel like going, wait for a couple of miles. And when you want to go again, wait for another couple of miles. Then, when you're ready again, wait for a couple more minutes.

— CHARLIE SPEDDING'S RUNNING ADVICE TO STEVE JONES

⬤

I remember watching Frank Shorter in the [1972 Munich Olympic] marathon. But I wasn't thinking that I'd end up in the Olympics. It was so far away from that, and something I couldn't conceive of.

— BILL RODGERS

Your body follows the directives of the mind. Racing is such a direct feedback system that whatever thoughts you are holding are immediately represented in your body.

— LORRAINE MOLLER

Doing something for yourself like running, and using it to test yourself, will only make you feel better about your career or your family role.

— JOAN BENOIT SAMUELSON

He runs like a man who's just been stabbed in the heart.

— A COACH ON EMIL ZATOPEK

⸻◆⸻

He runs with the grace of a bag thrown off the back of a mail truck. Somehow he finds the will to win.

— HAL HIGDON ON ALBERTO SALAZAR

⸻◆⸻

For me it's the same, altitude or not.

— SAID AOUITA ON TRAINING IN BOULDER, COLORADO

⸻◆⸻

Ahh, once I was entered, I tried to win. I came in second.

— EMIL ZATOPEK ON HIS FIRST RACE, WHICH HE TRIED TO GET OUT OF BY PLAYING SICK.

⸻◆⸻

Mr. Rodgers, you have to decide which is more important, your vocation or your avocation.

— School principal to Bill Rodgers

I've been trying to push it too far, but when you get to be 47 you start to think that time's not all before you, that you're not getting any younger, and there's a last-minute panic trying to cram everything in before the Big Curtain comes down.

— Priscilla Welch

He let the pack take him to 19 miles at perfect pace and he then found himself in the right place at the right time to move into the history books with an eyeballs-out, lung-busting, gut-wrenching six-mile surge to the finish.

— Charlie Spedding on Steve Jones's world record at the 1984 Chicago Marathon

They are the people I work with and get my hands dirty with. They could relate to me because I'm just Steve to them, not someone like Sebastian Coe or Steve Cram.

— STEVE JONES ON HIS FRIENDS AND COLLEAGUES

—◆—

The Boston Marathon was his solitary goal. He put everything he had into it.

— BILL RODGERS ON AMBY BURFOOT

—◆—

Numbers don't lie. You always seem to remember your workouts as being a little better than they were. It's good to go back and review what you do.

— FRANK SHORTER

—◆—

The fastest way from point A to point B is a constant pace.

— DAVE WELCH

———⊷∘⊶———

I wasn't concerned that Bill broke my American record. He ran a very good race at Boston. I was more concerned with my own training.

— FRANK SHORTER ON BILL RODGERS

———⊷∘⊶———

Keino had the biggest impact on the mile, because he was the one who really changed the way people were running. He came in at a time when pacing was thought to be the best way to run.

— MARTY LIQUORI ON HEZEKIAH KIPCHOGE "KIP" KEINO

———⊷∘⊶———

When Dad died, running was a release for me. I tend to store things inside me, and it's only when I go out for a run that I get it all out.

— STEVE JONES

———

Frank and Bill were both absolutely essential to the running boom, in completely different ways. Frank's biggest imprint was winning the Olympics. Frank was the Olympian in every sense, more regal, king of the land. Bill clearly was the boy next door.

— AMBY BURFOOT ON FRANK SHORTER AND BILL RODGERS

———

Bill found the formula that allowed him to recover quickly.

— FRANK SHORTER ON BILL RODGERS

———

After 10 years of tough marathon training, it was time to give the body a rest. I really was tired, and I needed to recoup. I needed to go back to 60 to 70 miles per week.

— PRISCILLA WELCH

Right now, I'm like I was in high school, just plugging along trying to run better, watching people run past me and telling myself, "Okay, next time I'll be a little closer, and maybe one day I'll be in front."

— FRANK SHORTER ON RUNNING AGAIN AFTER AN INJURY

All I was aware of was that Lisa was on my shoulder because I could hear her feet.

— LORRAINE MOLLER ON LISA MARTIN AT THE 1987 OSAKA MARATHON

I lost my anonymity forever.

— GRETE WAITZ ON THE CONSEQUENCES OF WINNING THE 1978
NEW YORK CITY MARATHON

<hr>

[Lorraine] runs like a race horse, and I mean that as a compliment. She has these loping strides.

— MARTY COOKSEY ON LORRAINE MOLLER

<hr>

[Y]ou never know what can happen during a jog around the block or a 5-mile run.

— FLORENCE GRIFFITH JOYNER

<hr>

Our ability to move for long distances at sub-maximal speeds is a gift to our species, like language.

— STU MITTLEMAN

I was just focused on the race. . . . It was just another race I was trying to do well in.

— BILL RODGERS ON THE 1975 BOSTON MARATHON, WHICH HE WON

I won't kid you and suggest that working out can't often seem like a chore, but I will tell you that the benefits far outweigh the sacrifice.

— FLORENCE GRIFFITH JOYNER

It sort of forces you to do it, because you don't want to let the other person down.

— GORDON BAKOULIS ON RUNNING WITH A PARTNER

My whole teaching in one sentence is: "Run slowly, run daily, drink moderately, and don't eat like a pig."

— DR. ERNEST VAN AAKEN, GERMAN PHYSICIAN AND RUNNING COACH

The average American takes twenty years to get out of condition and he wants to get back in condition in twenty days—and you just can't do it.

— DR. KEN COOPER

I get more gratification out of getting some obese person who had a heart attack running around and enjoying life within a year. I get more gratification from that than putting a person in the Olympic games.

— Arthur Lydiard

There is no doubt that "Sport for All" is a twentieth century movement of real significance. Other mass movements have oppressed where they intended to liberate. This movement liberates because it has an essentially individual basis. The choice of speed, route, distance, or company is entirely yours.

— Roger Bannister

I was tired from training and leading such a busy life, tired of having to bear the pressure and come through for others.

— Grete Waitz on her decision to reduce her running in 1976

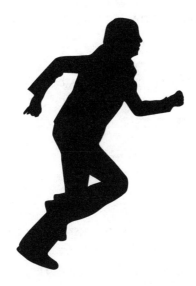

You may run faster tomorrow, but you won't run any bloody harder!

— Percy Cerutty

Fear is a great motivator.

— John Treacy

They stand near the line and pee on themselves. We always keep a mop near the start.

— FRED THOMPSON ON THE SIX-YEAR-OLDS AT THEIR FIRST
COMPETITION AT NEW YORK'S COLGATE GAMES

I better go home before he breaks the rest of my records.

— GUNDER HAGG, IN THE UNITED STATES, WHEN HE HEARD THAT
ARNE ANDERSSON HAD BROKEN HIS 1500M RECORD BACK IN SWEDEN

Charlie had foregone running for the money. I had won money, but it just happened. That's not what I went to Chicago for.

— STEVE JONES ON CHARLIE SPEDDING

I am very satisfied for now. . . . Please don't ask me about breaking 1:40!

— WILSON KIPKETER ON RUNNING 800 METERS IN 1:41.73, A NEW
RECORD

When Keino first came on the scene, he was the most flamboyant of the
early Kenyan runners.

— FRANK SHORTER ON HEZEKIAH KIPCHOGE "KIP" KEINO

"It is like a dream come true," I tell the journalists after the race. One
of them later writes that this seems too hackneyed to describe such an
emotional occasion. Well, what does he expect after a world record?
Shakespeare?

— BRENDAN FOSTER AFTER SETTING A 3000M WORLD RECORD

Dream barriers look very high until someone climbs them. Then they are not barriers anymore.

— LASSE VIREN

I'm afraid that record attempts are not in my line and this has strengthened my opposition to such a race.

— JACK LOVELOCK AFTER NOT SETTING A 1500M RECORD

Hills are the only beneficial type of resistance training for the runner.

— ARTHUR LYDIARD

God! He's running backwards!

> — BROADCASTER WHO SAW JIM PETERS COLLAPSE AT THE EMPIRE
> GAMES MARATHON IN 1954

⸺◆⸺

Great people and great athletes realize early in their lives their destiny, and accept it.

> — PERCY CERUTTY

⸺◆⸺

I ran to get a letter jacket, a girlfriend.

> — JIM RYUN

⸺◆⸺

My parents had a certain idea of what they wanted their little girl to be and it did not include a budding track star.

> — GRETE WAITZ

⸺◆⸺

When I was small I was very naughty and my father chased me with his belt to give me a thrashing. Maybe that was how I got accustomed to running.

— FERMIN CACHO

By a process of elimination, I went out for cross country.

— CLARENCE DeMAR

At my school, I was timekeeper. It was my responsibility to make sure the other students were on time. So it was important that I arrived always first.

— IBRAHAM HUSSEIN ON RUNNING MILES TO SCHOOL AS A CHILD IN KENYA

In those school races, I always ran my legs off. There were girls watching and I wanted to impress them.

— Juha Vaatainen

———◆———

I know my going into running with a vengeance was to have something clear, definable, and precise.

— Kenny Moore

———◆———

I am just an athlete who can get fit for the right race at the right time.

— Steve Jones

———◆———

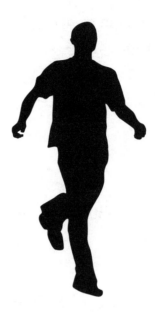

When I was 14 or 15, my brother tried to encourage me by giving me a pair of running shoes. But I threw them away because I was so used to running with bare feet and they were too heavy.

— HAILE GEBRSELASSIE

I lost my first race at school and I was so jealous when the winner received a puppet that I said to myself, "I will carry on until I win a puppet."

— SVETLANA MASTERKOVA

I look up to the five-minute milers. Because they don't get any of the good things I get. They're out there running just as hard.

— MARK BELGER

It was hard to find a pool when I was modeling in New York, so I took up running.

— KIM ALEXIS, SUPERMODEL

Sometimes people will say to me, "Oprah's got it easy because she's got a personal trainer and a personal chef." But that's baloney. No one can run for you. She was on the track every morning.

— BOB GREENE, OPRAH WINFREY'S PERSONAL TRAINER

Music is my life, but running allows me to appreciate the music of the outdoors.

— GAIL WILLIAMS, HORNPLAYER

In every little village in the world there are great potential champions who only need motivation, development, and good exercise evaluation.

— ARTHUR LYDIARD

The connection with the ferment of adolescence is a vital one for many runners. It certainly was for me.

— KENNY MOORE

⟞⟡⟝

If you want to tell something to an athlete, say it quickly and give no alternatives.

— PAAVO NURMI

⟞⟡⟝

I do give the athletes a relatively free rein and for good reason. One of my principles is "Don't overcoach."

— BILL BOWERMAN

⟞⟡⟝

We run every race together. We are the same person.

— TOSHIHIKO SEKO ON HIS DECEASED COACH, KIYOSHI NAKAMURA

———

I would scold them or beat them when they were lazy or disobedient. But I only did it for their own good.

— CHINESE COACH MA JUNREN

———

I have a dream. When I retire, I want to become an inn-keeper. Occasionally, I hope this day will arrive tomorrow.

— KARI SINKKONEN, FINNISH COACH

———

Bill Bowerman was, and is, and ever shall be a generous, ornery, profane, beatific, unyielding, antic, impenetrably complex Oregon original.

— KENNY MOORE

If the furnace is hot enough, it will burn anything.

— JOHN L. PARKER, JR., IN *ONCE A RUNNER*

All men and nations eat too much, and for this reason are not fit.

— PAAVO NURMI

It used to be that I'd eat to run—and the more I ran, the more I needed to eat. But now I run to eat. I love to eat.

— TOM FLEMING

I remember looking out the window and wondering what was out there and, now and then, I'd see a runner go by.

— LORRAINE MOLLER ON HER HOSPITALIZATION AS A CHILD

All I want to do is drink beer and train like an animal.

— ROD DIXON

I don't drink. I don't kiss girls. These things do an athlete in.

— SULEIMAN NYAMBUI

I am firmly of the impression that the athlete who indulges in an occasional glass of [beer] will, other things being equal, derive greater benefits thereby than the man who preserves and adheres to a rigid teetotalism.

— ALF SHRUBB

———◈———

My strength comes from my coach. Just as Alberto Salazar runs with God, I run with Coach Nakamura.

— TOSHIHIKO SEKO

———◈———

Listen to your body. Do not be a blind and deaf tenant.

— DR. GEORGE SHEEHAN

———◈———

Live like a clock.

— JUMBO ELLIOTT ON HOW RUNNERS SHOULD ARRANGE THEIR DAYS

I'd run from my house down two blocks and back and lie on the ground and die.

— JIM RYUN ON TRAINING WHEN HE WAS FIFTEEN

Most of my time is devoted to thinking and running.

— JUMA IKANGAA

Stupid, blind determination forced me on.

— PETER SNELL

Everything you do is based on the two runs a day.

— MARTY LIQUORI ON TRAINING FOR THE OLYMPICS

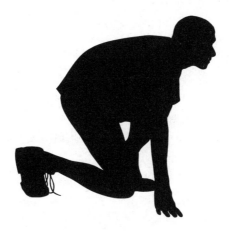

I think people can handle 150 to 200 miles a week. But something has to give somewhere.

— BILL BOWERMAN

＝◆＝

Some might say that it's easier to be the runner than the runner's family.

— ROBERT DE CASTELLA

＝◆＝

In my high school days, I found I couldn't defeat the other runners with speed, but I could on the distance side.

— BILL RODGERS

There is nothing more monotonous and sickening than running around a track.

— ARTHUR LYDIARD

All top international athletes wake up in the morning feeling tired and go to bed feeling very tired.

— BRENDAN FOSTER

There's a lot to be said for LSD—long, slow distance, in this case.

— JOE HENDERSON

I just want to make sure it's living hell for anyone out there who's going to beat me.

— KEN SOUZA ON WHY HE TRAINS SO HARD

———

When I was living on my father's farm I used to run over obstacles all the time, chasing the cows and sheep.

— MOSES KIPTAUNI ON HIS CHILDHOOD IN KENYA

———

[H]e may have been king of the roads, but he was not regal, not chilly.

— AMBY BURFOOT ON BILL RODGERS

———

I don't want to plead that it's the life of a monk, but I can't think of a sport—with the possible exception of swimming—where people train as hard.

— SEBASTIAN COE

The long run is what puts the tiger in the cat.

— BILL SQUIRES

I had no idea of speedwork, so it was no wonder I remained a slow trudger for so many years!

— PAAVO NURMI

I say I'm going to finish last. That takes the pressure off.

— DAN MIDDLEMAN

I found that working out in the morning helped get me going for the rest of the day, and working out in the afternoons helped relax me from a long day at the office.

— FLORENCE GRIFFITH JOYNER

If you want to win a race you have to go a little berserk.

— BILL RODGERS

Road racing is rock 'n roll; track is Carnegie Hall.

— MARTY LIQUORI

After 5 or 6 laps I have read everyone like a newspaper and I know who is able to do this or that.

— MIRUTS YIFTER

————————

I'm not a machine that can be wound up every day.

— HERB ELLIOTT

————————

I think the idea of a two-hour marathon is thoroughly ridiculous. Absolutely ridiculous.

— DEREK CLAYTON

————————

[D]on't be in a hurry, and never let any of the other runners know you are in a hurry even if you are.

— COLIN SMITH

———◆———

The struggle itself toward the heights is enough to fill man's heart. One must imagine Sisyphus happy.

— ALBERT CAMUS

———◆———

It is suicidal for other runners to copy my hill sessions without adequate backup.

— PEKKA VASALA

———◆———

The victory took the stamp of eccentricity off me. I was a real athlete. My running had been looked upon as a diversion before.

— FRANK SHORTER ON HIS 1972 OLYMPIC MARATHON WIN

———◆———

They are beautiful because they run and they run because they are beautiful.

— DR. ERNEST VAN AAKEN WHEN ASKED WHY BEAUTIFUL WOMEN RUN

———◆———

In a country where only men are encouraged, one must be one's own inspiration.

— TEGLA LOROUPE, KENYA

———◆———

You know, I'm no women's libber, but the media can really irritate me.
I sure get tired of being "pert" Francie Larrieu. That kind of stuff has to
stop. All those ridiculous adjectives they use with women.

— FRANCIE LARRIEU

A woman naturally thinks about how she looks, and the marathon beats
you up so much that you look terrible at the end. You do not happily
go before the camera. You just primp yourself as best you can and tell
yourself, well, what can I do about it?

— UTA PIPPIG

Joanie, if marathons make you look like this, please don't run anymore.

— JOAN BENOIT'S MOTHER IN A LETTER TO HER DAUGHTER AFTER
SEEING A PICTURE IN A NEWSPAPER

If this race is for "men only," why doesn't it say "men only" on the entry blank?

— NINA KUSCSIK IN 1969

People used to think I was a freak. Now women of all shapes and sizes run all the time. And they're not just beautiful and slim and wearing pink gossamer tights. They jiggle along at 12-minute miles or spring along at 6:30s. . . . That's what I love.

— KATHRINE SWITZER

New York is the one you have to win.

— ROD DIXON

I never felt as bad as I did over those last two miles. It was like running with a hangover.

— GEOFF SMITH ON THE 1983 NEW YORK MARATHON

I'm from Oregon, I hate New York, every day except Marathon Sunday.

— KENNY MOORE

Mind is everything: muscle—pieces of rubber. All that I am, I am because of my mind.

— PAAVO NURMI

If I ever did what he did, I'd be dead from sheer exhaustion.

— CHARLIE RODGERS ON HIS BROTHER BILL

———◆———

I don't know about psychology; I'm a runner.

— STEVE JONES

———◆———

The great thing about athletics is that it's like poker sometimes: you know what's in your hand and it may be a load of rubbish, but you've got to keep up the front.

— SEBASTIAN COE

———◆———

Running is in my blood—the adrenaline flows before the races, the love/ hate of butterflies in your stomach.

— MARCUS O'SULLIVAN

———◆———

I don't run for other people; I don't run for my country. I'm not very nationalistic. Derek Clayton comes first in my book.

— DEREK CLAYTON

———◆———

You could never get to talk to Nurmi. You could talk to the president of Finland, but not to Nurmi. He was a god.

— ARTHUR LYDIARD

———◆———

[The] frustrating aspect is that I still have to get permission to go to a race at which I might win $10,000 or $15,000, far more than I earn in a whole year with the RAF.

— STEVE JONES ON HIS DAY JOB

A being from another world.

— MICHEL JAZY ON HERB ELLIOTT

[Douglas Wakiihuri] has the legs of a Kenyan and the mind of a Japanese.

— JOHN TREACY

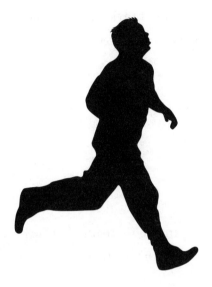

Top results are achieved only through pain. But eventually you like this pain.

— Juha Vaatainen

———◆———

Muscle has been grinding, sinew against bone—that's not like golf.

— Bill Rodgers

———◆———

At least in a race you have mile markers and know how long you have to go. Labor is like running as hard as you can without knowing where the finish line is.

— LORRAINE MOLLER ON CHILDBIRTH

The most important thing in the Olympic Games is not to win but to take part, just as the most important thing in life is not the triumph but the struggle.

— BARON DE COUBERTIN, FOUNDER OF THE MODERN OLYMPICS

You know, fourth is the absolutely worst place to finish in the Olympics.

— EAMONN COGHLAN

People claim that fourth is the worst place to finish in the Olympics or Olympic Trials. Maybe, but I finished fifth in one Olympic Trials, and I much rather would have finished fourth.

— HAL HIGDON

The Games are littered with people who had one good day and were never heard of or seen again.

— SEBASTIAN COE

Remember, to be second behind Herb Elliott is like being an Olympic Champion.

— MICHEL JAZY

Athletes should have the same opportunities as other artists and performers do, to perfect themselves through scholarships and fellowships to become artists in their sports.

— MARIO MONIZ PEREIRA, CARLOS LOPES'S COACH

We used to run just for the honor, for the glory, just to show people we could do it. The people run now because of the money involved, because of the contracts, because of the sponsors, etc.

— GASTON ROELANTS

Medals are nice, but they are only symbols.

— EMIL ZATOPEK

I would rather not race many times for just money; I would rather win little bits of metal at the end of a colored ribbon.

— CHARLES SPEDDING

If I had to choose between a gold medal and a happy family life, I'd take the good family life every time.

— RON CLARKE

There's a lot of pressure to keep my record sparkling—no silvers or bronzes.

— MICHAEL JOHNSON

I don't do it for the money. The minute you start focusing on the money, you lose sight of what you got into the sport for in the first place.

— KIM PAWELEK

——◆——

I compare it to a kid having a big jar of candy. At the beginning, you're stuffing your face with candy. Then, when you have only about a half-dozen pieces left, you start to savor them. You treat every race like it's special.

— MARCUS O'SULLIVAN ON THE END OF HIS RACING CAREER

——◆——

I can make a comeback if George Foreman can.

— SAID AOUITA

——◆——

The day I retire is the day they drop me into the fire or burn me.

— RON HILL

———⊰◆⊱———

Florence Griffith Joyner's contributions to society will undoubtedly last forever. Rarely do individuals possess the kind of strength, stability, and substance that took her from the ghetto of south-central Los Angeles to the White House in Washington, D.C.

— JACKIE JOYNER-KERSE ON FLORENCE GRIFFITH JOYNER

———⊰◆⊱———

Some people can't live without booze; it looks like I can't live without running.

— LASSE VIREN

———⊰◆⊱———

The athlete is another painter, another composer, another poet where the famous paintings, the sublime music, or the verses are replaced by world records. Athletics and running become a part of the story and tradition of the whole country in the future.

— GUNDER HAGG

If I faltered, there would be no arms to hold me and the world would be a cold and forbidding place.

— ROGER BANNISTER

It has such an historical significance, and it's such a big event, that, really, to win an Olympic medal for me is moving up into a new league. I'm in an exclusive club, something I have aspired to since I was a teenager.

— LORRAINE MOLLER

We can sprint the turn on a spring breeze and feel the winter leave our feet!

— Quentin Cassidy in John L. Parker Jr.'s *Once a Runner*

———◆———

If everybody could get in on [running] on a world scale, it would really be hard for people to go to war.

— Ron Daws

———◆———

It's just personal satisfaction.

— Kenny Moore

———◆———

What used to be just a simple break-neck run when I was a little girl turned into some pretty technical training that involved a great deal of mental effort.

— FLORENCE GRIFFITH JOYNER

I have to give up so many things, make so many personal sacrifices, to perform at my level, that I cannot even contemplate losing.

— SEBASTIAN COE

In the moment of victory I did not realize that the inner force, which had been driving me to my ultimate goal, died when I became the world's fastest miler.

— DEREK IBBOTSON IN 1957

He had enough sense to back off when he needed to, and also was able to take on a lot of work.

— CHARLIE RODGERS ON HIS BROTHER BILL

——⊰◈⊱——

It is very disappointing to lose in the last stride by the length of your nose.

— YEVGENY ARZHANOV

——⊰◈⊱——

Sometimes the difference between a good and a great runner is only an inch, as measured by exercise scientists. A good runner lifts two inches off the ground with each stride. A great runner rises only one inch, thus conserves energy.

— HAL HIGDON

——⊰◈⊱——

It was important for me to win this for Soh Kee-Chung, the hero of 1936. It was also for my mother who during the entire race was at the temple praying that I would win the gold for Korea.

— HWANG YOUNG-JO, 1992 WINNER OF THE OLYMPIC MARATHON

The Australian behavior toward losers is far from healthy. If youngsters are taught that losing is a disgrace, and if they're not sure they can win, they will be reluctant to even try. And not trying is the real disgrace.

— RON CLARKE

Just as I always dreamed in secret, I raised my arms, I smiled, and I crossed the finish line.

— JOSY BARTHEL

I had improved my fitness a big chunk. It was great fun, and winning Boston changed my life.

— BILL RODGERS ON THE 1975 BOSTON MARATHON

Three hours slow is better than two hours fast.

— PETE GAVUZZI, COACH TO GERARD COTE

Over the years much has changed in my life, but my focus on running has remained consistently strong.

— JOAN BENOIT SAMUELSON

When I started running and competing at the age of 7, I had the worst form of anyone else running, and my coaches told me that if I wanted to improve my times, I had to improve my running form.

— FLORENCE GRIFFITH JOYNER

Bill was able to run a lot of races at a high level. I can think of only three runners who were able to do that: Bill, Juma Ikangaa, and Doug Kurtis.

— FRANK SHORTER ON BILL RODGERS

We didn't learn about anaerobic thresholds—simply the joy of running.

— AMBY BURFOOT ON JOHN KELLEY

As long as I run, I will always lift weights. To me, running without weight training is like running barefoot because something so valuable is missing.

— FLORENCE GRIFFITH JOYNER

———⟨◆⟩———

The challenge and the energy running requires may be a selfish one, but it actually motivates me to be stronger in my relationships.

— JOAN BENOIT SAMUELSON

———⟨◆⟩———

The Olympics are a dinosaur, running out of cities. . . . If you use the politics of a nation to judge whether or not you compete with that nation, you might as well say that international sport is dead.

— SEBASTIAN COE

———⟨◆⟩———

If track is serious about ridding the sport of illegal drugs, then a separate organization is needed, whose only duty is to catch cheaters, regardless of the potential media impact.

— STEVE HOLMAN

Hitler was there every day, watching. He looked like Charlie Chaplin sitting up there, him and that fat guy, Goering.

— JOHN A. KELLY, ON THE 1936 BERLIN OLYMPICS

Thrust against pain, pain is the purifier.

— PERCY CERUTTY

When I am running, I feel everything is in sync. Even my mechanical leg becomes a part of me.

— SARAH REINERSTEN

Concentration is why some athletes are better than others. You develop that concentration in training. You can't be lackadaisical in training and concentrate in a meet.

— EDWIN MOSES

I love buying running shoes. I don't mean that I just enjoy the process of trying on new shoes. I mean I love buying running shoes.

— JOHN BINGHAM

By breaking the world record every few days, those two Limeys are making a mockery of the mile race, which has traditionally been the core and kernel of any track meet.

— RED SMITH, REFERRING TO SEBASTIAN COE AND STEVE OVETT

The body does not want you to do this. As you run, it tells you to stop but the mind must be strong. You always go too far for your body. You must handle the pain with strategy. It is not age; it is not diet. It is the will to succeed.

— JACQUELINE GAREAU

CHAPTER FIVE

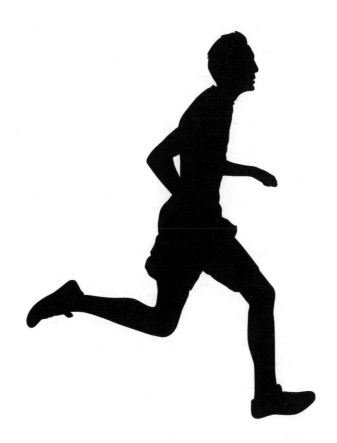

They said it on a T-shirt

Fleeting Thoughts

"Fartlek." That was the word on the shirt of a woman running near me in a road race. And on her back, the half-explanation: "It's a runner's thing."

That serves as my favorite quote on a T-shirt, but it takes some explanation if you don't know your running history. The world's two fastest milers in the 1940's were Swedes: Gunder Hagg and Arne Anderson. Much of the rest of the world then was at war, but not Sweden. Hagg's coach at that time was Gosta Holmer, who devised a form of training called "fartlek." The word translated loosely as "speedplay" and described a free form of training where you ran in the woods, alternating fast and slow runs of no particular distance, training intuitively.

That's a mouthful to put on the back of a t-shirt. Better to say, "It's a runner's thing."

T-shirts proliferate at high school cross-country meets, each team seemingly seeking to outdo the other in backside mottos. That includes my home town: Michigan City High School. Each year a new t-shirt; each year a new slogan. The best recent one on the back of City runners: "In this life there are leaders and followers. Take note: You are reading the back of my shirt."

Great runners deserve great T-shirts. Perhaps one or more of the quotes in this chapter will wind up soon on the back of a runner near you.

My therapist is the pavement. My drug is endorphins. My foe is the next hill. I am a runner.

Feet don't fail me now.

Running a marathon is 90 percent mental toughness. The rest is in your head.

I run, therefore I am.

My lunch hours aren't for eating, my Saturday mornings aren't for sleeping, and my holidays aren't for taking it easy. I am a runner.

I'm the fast girl your mother warned you about.

May the course be with you.

Everyone gets knocked down. Champions get up.

Running is a mental sport and we're all insane.

Trample the weak. Hurdle the dead.

A Marathoner's Response:
Yes, it's REALLY hard
Yes, I had to train A LOT
Yes, I know it's HARD on the body
Yes, I know I'm CRAZY and . . .

It's funner with a runner.

Train hard, win easy.

Run, eat, sleep. Repeat.

In a world of give and take, give what it takes.

There is no bench in cross-country.

Run hard when it's hard to run.

Got lactic acid?

Stand still and life will pass you by . . . Run!

Runners don't die; they only smell like it.

Kiss my Asics!

We eat miles for breakfast

Like my back? You'll be seeing a lot more of it.

My cross-country shoes have more miles than your car!

Run with the best . . . dust for the rest.

Our mascara runs faster than you.

If cross-country were easy it would be called football.

Summer miles bring autumn smiles!

Cross-country runners do it in the woods.

Dream BIG, Run fast!!!

I run because I like to; I win because I have to

Running Begins Not With the Feet But With the Mind

If you can read this, you should give up now.

Whoever said it's not whether you win or lose that count's . . . probably LOST!!

You ask me why I run? The same reason I breathe, I have to!

How does my butt look like from back there?

Running is my girlfriend

Everyone looks up at the stars in the sky, but a champion climbs a mountain and gets one.

Girl's Cross Country: you don't need balls to do it.

Rage against the course.

Live to run . . . run to live!

If I'm not limping, it's because both sides hurt.

CHAPTER SIX

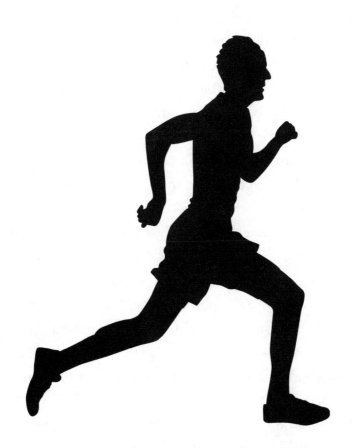

Triumph and tragedy

Running Races

All my marathon training programs peak at 20 miles. And among the most frequently asked questions asked me at lectures or posted to the bulletin boards I manage online is: "How can I expect to run 26 miles 385 yards when the furthest you let me run in practice is 20 miles?"

My glib answer is to suggest that a quarter-million runners using my programs have taken that approach. "Have faith," I say.

But the truth is that before a marathon, or any other important race, runners will have rested. For a marathon, they taper three weeks. Even an important 5-K requires a cutback in training for three or four days if you expect to do your best. In contrast, that 20-mile run is completed after a hard week of work.

Before a race, runners eat right. They skip that extra beer or glass of wine the night before. They don't stay out late. They get to sleep early. When they step to the starting line the next morning, it is with a purpose, more than for just another day in practice. Once moving, the sounds of the crowd and the footsteps of their fellow competitors carry them along. Several top athletes quoted in this chapter talk about the "fear" of failure. I have never been able to run as fast in practice as I have in either a track meet or road race.

As for the marathon and why I recommend a longest run of only 20 miles, I consider the last 6 miles 385 yards to be sacred ground. You only dare enter with a number pinned to your chest.

Do otherwise, and the gods will be angry.

No matter how old I get, the race remains one of life's most rewarding experiences.

— GEORGE SHEEHAN

———◦———

My thoughts before a big race are usually pretty simple. I tell myself: "Get out of the blocks, run your race, stay relaxed. If you run your race, you'll win. . . . Channel your energy. Focus."

— CARL LEWIS

———◦———

You hear it over and over again—a television announcer saying, "Watch that guy, he looks so relaxed." It's a rare athlete who wins who doesn't look relaxed.

— MARK ALLEN

———◦———

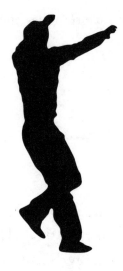

The longer the race, the shorter the champ.

— 10KTRUTH.COM

❖

I was unable to walk for a whole week after that, so much did the race take out of me. But it was the most pleasant exhaustion I have ever known.

— EMIL ZATOPEK ON HIS MARATHON WIN AT THE HELSINKI OLYMPICS

❖

When you put yourself on the line in a race and expose yourself to the unknown, you learn things about yourself that are very exciting.

— DORIS BROWN HERITAGE

A road race is the closest thing to a party I can think of.

— BILL RODGERS, *BILL RODGERS' LIFETIME RUNNING PLAN*

There will come a point in the race, when you alone will need to decide. You will need to make a choice. Do you really want it? You will need to decide.

— ROLF ARANDS

The possibilities in racing tactics are almost unlimited, as in a game of chess, for every move there is a counter, for every attack there is a defense.

— FRANZ STAMPFL, *FRANZ STAMPFL ON RUNNING*

I train to race. I love to train, but I love to race even more.

— LYNN JENNINGS

A slight hesitance, a single step to the inside, a few seconds miscalculation of the right pace of the timing of the final kick, and any other seemingly minor error, may throw away months and years of careful preparation and sacrifice.

— KEN DOHERTY

Good health, peace of mind, being outdoors, camaraderie—those are all wonderful things that come to you when running. But for me, the real pull of running—the proverbial icing on the cake—has always been racing.

— BILL RODGERS, *BILL RODGERS' LIFETIME RUNNING PLAN*

There is a world of difference between racing for time and racing to win. The white line and clear course are needed for one; generalship, ability to change pace, and track tactics for the other.

— THE *DAILY MIRROR*, JUNE 4, 1954

Some runners judge performance by whether they won or lost. Others define success or failure by how fast they ran. Only you can judge your performance. Avoid letting others sit in judgment of you.

— HAL HIGDON

Sex doesn't always determine who will be the fastest. . . . Look at any race and you'll see that the best women beat most of the men.

— CLAIRE KOWALCHIK, *THE COMPLETE BOOK OF RUNNING FOR WOMEN*

To make your life a work of art, you must have the material to work with. The race, any race, is just such an experience.

— GEORGE SHEEHAN

No one competes with the reckless abandon they should. . . . I'd personally rather watch someone who runs his guts out, throws his breakfast up and passes out at the end of the race.

— JOHN SCHIEFER

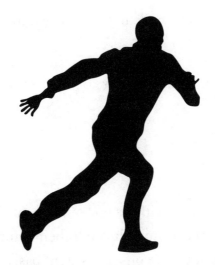

Why run a race? You race to test yourself, for the ritual, the camaraderie, and for the adventure and discovery.

— *THE NEW YORK ROAD RUNNERS CLUB COMPLETE BOOK OF RUNNING*

The man who can drive himself further once the effort gets painful is the man who will win.

— ROGER BANNISTER

Most mistakes in a race are made in the first two minutes, perhaps in the very first minute.

— Jack Daniels, Exercise Physiologist and Coach

Average runners often use racing as one of the goals in their training. Maybe it is to help them continue through their training, maybe it motivates them to get out there on a consistent basis.

— Frank Shorter

You should not do more than two races a month if you want those races to be key, maximum efforts. . . . Otherwise, staleness and breakdown may occur.

— Cliff Held

I tell my athletes, "When you compete, concentrate on yourself. Don't focus on anger against a competitor."

— JOE DOUGLAS

When we stop this nonsense of running like a metronome and with the watch always in mind, we will get back to real racing, the triumph of one runner over another. That is what racing was meant to be and what it will be when we get the four-minute myth out of the way.

— COLONEL STRODE JACKSON, 1912 OLYMPIC 1,500-METER CHAMPION

There's nothing graceful about it. You don't start where you finish, it's ugly.

— JOHN LANDY ON THE 1,500 METER RACE

I shall learn to have a better style once they start judging races according to their beauty. So long as it's a question of speed then my attention will be directed to seeing how fast I can cover the ground.

— EMIL ZATOPEK ON HIS RUNNING STYLE

To be consistently good, once you're in your own lane, you run your own race. For racing, this is the best way to take your nervous energy and turn it into positive energy.

— JOE DOUGLAS

Racing is pain, and that's why you do it, to challenge yourself and the limits of your physical and mental barriers. You don't experience that in an armchair watching television.

— MARK ALLEN

Even if you're not racing seriously, it pays to choose a well-organized race with a good reputation.

— *THE NEW YORK ROAD RUNNERS CLUB COMPLETE BOOK OF RUNNING*

I look at victory as milestones on a very long highway.

— JOAN BENOIT SAMUELSON

Racing entails risk. The most common mistake in addition to overtraining is racing too much too soon.

— TOM FLEMING

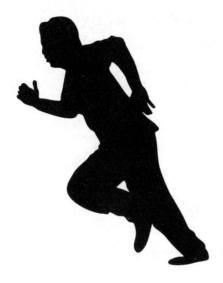

If I do well in a race I'm to the moon. If I do exceptionally well, I've jumped over that moon.

— PRISCILLA WELCH

�⟩

To avoid starting out too fast, you have to "have eyes in your stomach," as we say in Norwegian: a good gut instinct of control.

— GRETE WAITZ

This is a game of winning and losing. It is senseless to explain and explain.

— PAAVO NURMI

You can walk during a race if you wish.

— BOB GLOVER, *THE RUNNER'S HANDBOOK*

The difference between a jogger and a runner is an entry blank.

— GEORGE SHEEHAN

Everyone in life is looking for a certain rush. Racing is where I get mine.

— JOHN TRAUTMANN

Inevitably, there's some official bellowing: "Come on! Run through the chute! Keep it movin'!" But you're bent over, gasping, admiring with salt-stung eyes the good, honest mud of battle . . . splattered on your still-quivering legs and too-old (but still lucky) racing shoes. What could be more beautiful?

— MARK WILL-WEBER

My whole feeling in terms of racing is that you have to be very bold. You sometimes have to be aggressive and gamble.

— BILL RODGERS

The agony of the runners was a visible, tangible thing. It was only courage and the deepest reserves of stamina that were driving them round the track, still competing, still fighting it out.

— WILLIAM R. LOADER, "STAYING THE DISTANCE"

There is something about the ritual of the race—putting on the number, lining up, being timed—that brings out the best in us.

— GRETE WAITZ

———✦———

Fear is probably the thing that limits performance more than anything— the fear of not doing well, of what people will say. You've got to acknowledge those fears, then release them.

— MARK ALLEN

———✦———

Foley knew the dread of the slow minutes before a race begins—the draw for the positions, the bumbling instructions from judge and starter, the final hush when the starter's commands begin: "On your marks!"

— EDDY ORCUTT, "WHEELBARROW"

———✦———

[I]n athletics, the main essence is races, races against opponents, more than against the clock. . . . And those will be what I shall set my main sights on.

— ROGER BANNISTER

I'm going to go and leave my blood all over the track.

— NICK ROGERS, OLYMPIAN

I made the school team, and when I won in a match against another school it was the greatest moment of my life—even greater than the European titles. In those school races, I always ran my legs off. There were girls watching and I wanted to impress them. I was foaming and vomiting, but I won.

— JUHA VÄÄTÄINEN

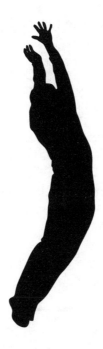

I don't understand why members of the media have to try so hard for stories. For real fans, the events speak for themselves as well as the performances and the corresponding drama. Excitement in track and field does not come from heartbreaking stories. It is in the competition and the buildup.

— JOHN SCHIEFER

It wasn't enough for me to win the race. I wanted to bury the other guys.

— ALBERTO SALAZAR

In the field of sports, you are more or less accepted for what you do rather than what you are.

— ALTHEA GIBSON

Strategy-wise, go with your strengths. If you don't have a great finish, you must get away to win.

— JOHN TREACY

I love controlling a race, chewing up an opponent. Let's get down and dirty. Let's fight it out. It's raw, animalistic, with no one to rely on but yourself. There's no better feeling than that.

— ADAM GOUCHER, WINNER 1999 US NATIONALS 5000 TITLE

While a man is racing he must hate himself and his competitors.

— PERCY CERUTTY

A race is a work of art that people can look at and be affected by in as many ways as they're capable of understanding.

— STEVE PREFONTAINE

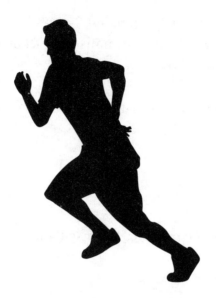

In any race there are the moments you feel great, and the moments you feel you're not going to make it.

— MARK ALLEN

You have your own strategy and what you do is go out and use it, and structure the situation so everyone else is forced to use your strategy . . . it really is a control issue.

— FRANK SHORTER

The ambition of the runners of the English aristocracy was to beat the horses in speed. Many instances might be cited of their having wagered that they would beat a team of horses, and however surprising it may seem, of their winning the bets.

— CHARLES RUSSELL

The only tactics I admire are do-or-die.

— HERB ELLIOTT

First is first, and second is nowhere.

— IAN STEWART

Thank God, it's over.

— NEIL CUSACK, 1974 MARATHON WINNER

I felt my throat start to close up, and I didn't think I was getting enough oxygen. I was scared, and I thought about quitting. But you don't want to quit when you've trained so hard and long for one race.

— DEENA DROSSIN DESCRIBING THE EFFECTS OF BEING STUNG BY A BEE IN THE BACK OF THE THROAT 100 METERS AFTER THE START OF THE WORLD CROSS-COUNTRY CHAMPIONSHIPS IN PORTUGAL. DESPITE BLACKING OUT AND FALLING DURING THE 8K RACE, SHE FINISHED IN TWELFTH PLACE.

———◦—◦———

The most challenging aspect of the decathlon is not the events themselves, but how you train to become the best 100-meter runner you are on the same day that you're the best 1,500-meter runner.

— BRUCE JENNER

———◦—◦———

My times become slower and slower, but the experience of the race is unchanged: each race a drama, each race a challenge, each race stretching me in one way or another, and each race telling me more about myself and others.

— GEORGE SHEEHAN

If you can't win, make the fellow ahead of you break the record.

— UNKNOWN

The single biggest change in middle-distance running, from the 1500 meters to 10,000 meters, has been the track surface.

— HERB ELLIOTT

A lesser but still fundamental rule of racing is that you properly enter the event. Anyone who doesn't but still insists on running interferes with the paying customers.

— JOE HENDERSON

Second place is not a defeat. It is a stimulation to get better. It makes you even more determined.

— CARLOS LOPES

Only think of two things—the gun and the tape. When you hear the one, just run like hell until you break the other.

— SAM MUSSABINI

A race is a breed apart from the daily run.

— GAIL W. KISLEVITZ

The thin line of worsted at the finish was almost within grasping distance. The two athletes were reeling under the cruelty of it all. It was horribly wrong that one of them should have to lose.

— WILLIAM R. LOADER, "STAYING THE DISTANCE"

I much prefer racing against men than against the clock. It is much more fun.

— CHRIS CHATAWAY

When I did this three years ago, it was like death. When I did it last year, it was like near-death. This year, it was just really hard.

— JOHN HOWIE, WHEELCHAIR ATHLETE, ON HIS CHARLOTTE OBSERVER 10K RACES

Running became boring because it's so predictable. I got to a point where I knew what my competition could do.

— PETER SNELL

I know it's going to be difficult. You just hope that you have the perfect day. What else can I do, sit home? You go out there to race. If you've got the qualifying mark, you've got to go out there.

— RYAN SHAY, ON THE 2008 U.S. MEN'S OLYMPIC MARATHON TRIALS,
DURING WHICH HE COLLAPSED AND DIED

The thing that made him such a great runner may have killed.

— JOE SHAY, ON THE DEATH OF HIS SON RYAN, WHO HAD BEEN
DIAGNOSED WITH AN ENLARGED HEART, WHICH MIGHT HAVE GIVEN
HIM EXTRA ENDURANCE

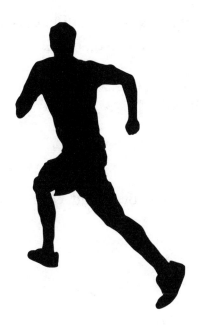

We told our guys to hold on for thirty minutes of agony for twelve months of glory.

— JOHN MCDONNELL, COACH OF ARKANSAS, WHICH WON THE 1993 NCAA CROSS-COUNTRY TITLE

I prefer running without shoes. My toes didn't get cold. Besides, if I'm in front from the start, no one can step on them.

— MICHELLE DEKKERS, THE BAREFOOT SOUTH AFRICAN RUNNER WHO WON THE 1989 NCAA CROSS-COUNTRY TITLE FOR INDIANA

A running machine that glides over mud, crud, and goop.

— ED EYESTONE ON JOHN NGUGI

The secret of cross-country is to do everything we do on the track and take it into the bush.

— MIKE KOSKEI, FORMER NATIONAL COACH OF KENYA

The crime is not to avoid failure, the crime is to not give triumph a chance.

— H. WELDON

Blink and you miss a sprint. The 10,000 meters is lap after lap of waiting. Theatrically, the mile is just the right length—beginning, middle, end: a story unfolding.

— Sebastian Coe

Some of the world's greatest feats were accomplished by people not smart enough to know they were impossible.

— Doug Larson

If you want to race and get the best possible results, choose races carefully and focus on them.

— Francie Larrieu Smith

Get out well, but not too quickly, move through the field, be comfortable.

— JOHN TREACY

———◆———

It made him more mentally fit to compete when he ran. It strengthened his will; his inner discipline.

— RICHARD CHRISTIAN MATHESON, "THIRD WIND"

———◆———

If you don't try to win, you might as well hold the Olympics in somebody's backyard.

— JESSE OWENS

———◆———

If you want to win anything—a race, yourself, your life—you have to go a little berserk.

— GEORGE SHEEHAN

———◆———

Often I visualize a quicker, almost like a ghost runner, ahead of me with a quicker stride. It's really crazy. In races, this always happens to me.

— GABE JENNINGS

I prefer to remain in blissful ignorance of the opposition. That way I'm not frightened by anyone's reputation.

— IAN THOMPSON

I tell our runners to divide the race into thirds. Run the first part with your head, the middle part with your personality, and the last part with your heart.

— MIKE FANELLI, COACH

No negative thoughts cross my mind on race day. When I look into their eyes, I know I'm going to beat them.

— DANNY HARRIS

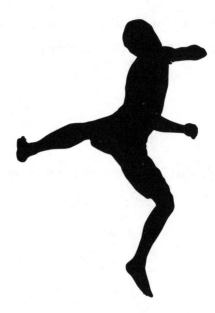

The will to win means nothing if you haven't the will to prepare.

— JUMA IKANGAA

Once you have decided that winning isn't everything, you become a winner.

— GEORGE SHEEHAN

For I have lost the race I never ran,
A rathe December blights my lagging May

— HARTLEY COLERIDGE, "LONG TIME A CHILD"

After a while, if you feel good, pick up your pace. Start picking off runners; you're the tortoise passing the hares who went too fast.

— BOB GLOVER AND SHELLY-LYNN FLORENCE GLOVER, *THE COMPETITIVE RUNNER'S HANDBOOK*

I'm a competitor. I really enjoyed the race more than just going out and running to run.

— SHANNON MILLER

I've won some big races and I've had some big disappointments.

— ALBERTO SALAZAR

If I lose forcing the pace all the way, well, at least I can live with myself.

— STEVE PREFONTAINE

Nothing splendid has ever been achieved except by those who dared believe that something inside them was superior to circumstance.

— BILL BARTON

I never race at all; I just run, and somehow I know that if I forget I'm racing and only jog-trot alog until I don't know I'm running I always win the race.

— ALAN SILLITOE, "THE LONELINESS OF THE LONG-DISTANCE RUNNER"

I don't want to lose to no one.

— GABE JENNINGS

⟐

I ran my first sub-4-minute mile in 1977 and since then have run 136 more. Nobody has run as many sub-4s as I have, and I intend to run at least one more.

— STEVE SCOTT, AFTER CANCER SURGERY

⟐

The 800-meter record, the records in the 1000, the 1500, the 5000, the relays: no one remembers them. The mile, they remember. Only the mile.

— JOHN WALKER

⟐

The mile has all the elements of drama.

— ROGER BANNISTER

⟞◆⟝

Almost every part of the mile is tactically important: you can never let down, never stop thinking, and you can be beaten at almost any point. I suppose you could say it is like life.

— JOHN LANDY

⟞◆⟝

I've always found it effective to make a move just before the crest of a hill. You get away just a little and you're gone before your opponent gets over the top.

— JOHN TREACY

⟞◆⟝

If there are five people of equal abilities, it is just who can compete in the situation in such a way that makes everyone pursue the event at that moment in the way that most suits you.

— FRANK SHORTER

A starting line is the best, most exciting place I can imagine.

— AMBY BURFOOT, *THE RUNNER'S GUIDE TO THE MEANING OF LIFE*

Roger Bannister studied the four-minute mile the way Jonas Salk studied polio—with a view to eradicating.

— JIM MURRAY, *LOS ANGELES TIMES* COLUMNIST

Winning breeds winning. Losing breeds losing, and when you're losing, you don't think of anything else.

— ANGELINA WOLVERT

To boast of a performance which I cannot beat is merely stupid vanity. And if I can beat it that means there is nothing special about it.

— EMIL ZATOPEK

If you don't have confidence, you'll always find a way not to win.

— CARL LEWIS

He does everything wrong but win.

— LARRY SNYDER, OHIO STATE TRACK COACH, ON EMIL ZATOPEK'S RUNNING STYLE

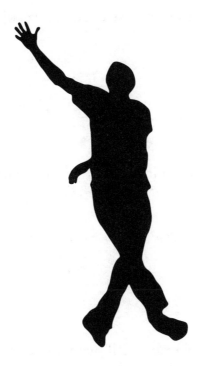

Just remember this: no one ever won the olive wreath with an impressive training diary.

— MARTY LIQUORI

Three failures denote uncommon strength. A weakling has not enough grit to fail thrice.

— MINNA THOMAS ANTRIM

———◆———

The gun goes off and everything changes . . . the world changes . . . and nothing else really matters.

— PATTI SUE PLUMMER

———◆———

When people ask me why I run, I tell them, there's not really a reason, it's just the adrenaline when you start, and the feeling when you cross that finish line, and know that you are a winner no matter what place you got.

— COURTNEY PARSONS

———◆———

Jogging through the forest is pleasant, as is relaxing by the fire with a glass of gentle Bordeaux and discussing one's travels. Racing is another matter. The frontrunner's mind is filled with an anguished fearfulness, a panic, which drives into pain.

— KENNY MOORE

No one knows the fear in a frontrunner's mind more than me. When you set off at a cracking pace for four or five laps and find that your main rivals are still breathing down your neck, that's when you start to panic.

— RON CLARKE

He cleared the hurdles like he feared they had spikes imbedded on the top, and leaped the water hazard as if he thought crocodiles were swimming in it.

— DESCRIPTION OF KENYA'S AMOS BIWOTTS

I thought I was back to a normal state until somebody summoned me to the starting line. It was like feeling a blade go through my flesh.

— JULES LADOUMEGUE

When the meal was over we all had a quiet rest in our rooms and I meditated on the race. This is the time when an athlete feels all alone in the big world.

— GORDON PIRIE

Fear is the strongest driving-force in competition. Not fear of one's opponent, but of the skill and high standard which he represents; fear, too, of not acquitting oneself well.

— FRANZ STAMPFL

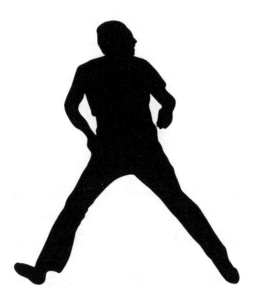

I saw over 100,000 people in the stands, and before I knew it, I had collapsed onto the infield grass. . . . I guess the humor of that image made me lose my nervousness. I was able to recover, get up and jog to the starting line.

— TOM COURTNEY, GOLD MEDAL WINNER OF THE 800M IN MELBOURNE

The mile has a classic symmetry. It's a play in four acts.

— JOHN LANDY

The 10,000 meters is lap after lap of waiting.

— SEBASTIAN COE

There was nothing unusual about my victory. The entire story was back in eighth place. There is simply no way to imagine how good Jim Ryun is or how far he will go after he becomes an adult.

— DYROL BURLESON, AFTER WINNING THE COMPTON INVITATIONAL MILE ON JUNE 5TH, 1964. RYUN, JUST 17, RAN 3.59.0

I have never been a killer. I'm not an aggressive personality and if I can remember any emotion I felt during a race it was fear. The greatest stimulator of my running was fear.

— HERB ELLIOTT

Opponents assume tremendous stature. Any runner who denies having fears, nerves or some kind of disposition is a bad athlete, or a liar.

— GORDON PIRIE

The new Kenyans. There are always new Kenyans.

— NOUREDDINE MORCELLI, WHEN ASKED IF HE FEARED ANY OTHER RUNNERS

Big occasions and races which have been eagerly anticipated almost to the point of dread, are where great deeds can be accomplished.

— JACK LOVELOCK

In the achievement of greater performances, of beating formidable rivals, the athlete defeats fear and conquers himself.

— FRANZ STAMPFL

I eat whatever the guy who beat me in the last race ate.

— ALEX RATELLE

———◆———

Whether we athletes liked it or not, the 4-minute mile had become rather like an Everest: a challenge to the human spirit, it was a barrier that seemed to defy all attempts to break it, an irksome reminder that men's striving might be in vain.

— ROGER BANNISTER

———◆———

The athlete knows he controls what happens to him. He blames no one but himself when things go wrong.

— GEORGE SHEEHAN

———◆———

As soon as I was in front I started praying for someone to pass me. It was a horrible realization. . . . Instead of running it out of them, I was running it out of me.

— EAMONN COGHLAN

I used very, very poor judgment and I'm man enough to admit that.

— JOHN A. KELLY, AFTER PRESSING TOO EARLY IN A RACE TO ELLISON BROWN, WHO EVENTUALLY BEAT HIM WITH AN UNEXCEPTIONAL TIME.

You've got fast feet. But there are millions of people who have fast feet. The people who win races are the ones with fast brains.

— ROSS KITT, FATHER OF A.J. KITT, TO KITT BEFORE A A BIG RACE

I haven't run as fast as I can, I haven't spoken as well as I can, and I haven't written as well as I can. If you take any less than that view, you're finished.

— GEORGE SHEEHAN

These high, wild hills and rough, uneven ways draw out our miles and make them wearisome.

— SHAKESPEARE, *RICHARD II*

I'd rather run a gutsy race, pushing all the way and lose, than run a conservative race only for a win.

— ALBERTO SALAZAR

You have to forget your last marathon before you try another. Your mind can't know what's coming.

— FRANK SHORTER

———◆———

Everyone stumbles at one time or another. It's the human condition.

— AMBY BURFOOT, *THE RUNNER'S GUIDE TO THE MEANING OF LIFE*

———◆———

Several times I have been threatened with overthrow by phenomenals. On one or two occasions it has been whispered around in such a way as to reach my ears, that importations have been made and it was goodbye to Shrubb. These importations have once or twice materialized. Like deer they would run for a distance and keep me guessing. All of a sudden they would disappear and I, smilingly relieved, would trudge on alone.

— ALF SHRUBB

———◆———

CHAPTER SEVEN

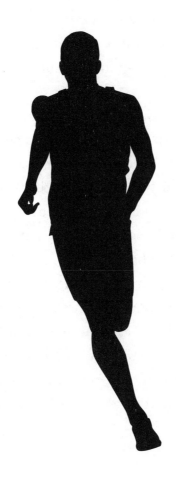

Writers on running

Running in Literature

Most non-runners know the term "the loneliness of the long distance runner," even if they have not seen the 1962 film by that name, nor read the short story by Alan Sillitoe on which it is based. Non-runners sometimes interpret this to mean that running is a solitary pursuit, thus no fun.

But the hero in the film, Colin Smith, sent to a boy's reformatory after being caught burglarizing a bakery, finds peace through running. It becomes Smith's escape. When allowed to run in the woods to train for a cross-country race, he finds the time spent running alone to be the most pleasurable moments of his otherwise dreary day. "I ran to a steady jog-trot rhythm, and soon it was so smooth that I forgot I was running," writes Sillitoe in the voice of his runner.

Most of us can identify with that feeling, though probably we would not act as Sillitoe's runner did in the story's climactic moment: stopping a few strides from the finish line, taunting his coach and those who had cheered him, refusing to cross the line and win the race.

Still, literature can bring us to lines we can never cross. Such is the loneliness of the long distance reader, and it is not unpleasant.

Great Akhilleus, hard on Hektor's heels,
kept after him, the way a hound will harry
a deer's fawn he has startled from its bed
to chase through gorge and open glade, and when
the quarry goes to earth under a bush
he holds the scent and quarters till he finds it;
so with Hektor: he could not shake off
the great runner, Akhilleus.

— HOMER, *THE ILIAD*

———◆———

I listened to the rhythm of my breath, which was unsteady as early as twelve miles into the race. By fifteen miles, lots of women were passing me and I understood that I might not make it. Without despair I continued step by step.

— MAX APPLE, "CARBO-LOADING"

———◆———

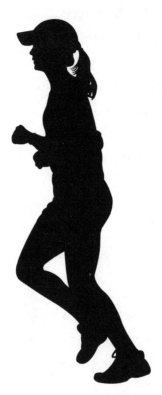

"Would you—be good enough—"Alice panted out, after running a little further, "to stop a minute—just to get—one's breath again?"
"I'm good enough," the King said, "only I'm not strong enough. You see, a minute goes by so fearfully quick. You might as well try to stop a Bandersnatch!"

— LEWIS CARROLL, *THROUGH THE LOOKING-GLASS*

Out came the children running.
All the little boys and girls,
With rosy cheeks and flaxen curls,
And sparkling eyes and teeth like pearls,
Tripping and skipping, ran merrily after
The wonderful music with shouting and laughter.

— ROBERT BROWNING, "THE PIED PIPER OF HAMELIN"

Still as they run they look behind,
They hear a voice in every wind,
And snatch a fearful joy.

— THOMAS GRAY, "ODE ON A DISTANT PROSPECT OF ETON COLLEGE"

It was far in the sameness of the wood;
I was running with joy on the Demon's trail,
Though I knew what I hunted was no true god.

— ROBERT FROST, "THE DEMIURGE'S LAUGH"

If you can force your heart and nerve and sinew
To serve your turn long after they are gone,
And so hold on when there is nothing in you
Except the Will which says to them: "Hold on!"

— RUDYARD KIPLING, "IF"

The wind is old and still at play
While I must hurry upon my way,
For I am running to Paradise;
Yet never have I lit on a friend
To take my fancy like the wind
That nobody can buy or bind.

— WILLIAM BUTLER YEATS, "RUNNING TO PARADISE"

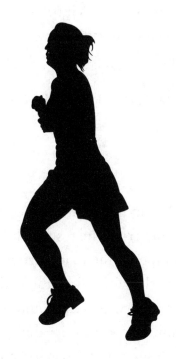

Achilles had strapped the wind
About his ankles,
He brushed rocks
The waves had flung.
He ran in armor.

— HILDA DOOLITTLE, "CHORUS OF THE WOMEN OF CHALKIS"

John Sobieski could see his own shoes hitting the sidewalk one after the other, while he himself seemed to ride above somewhere on some funny kind of running machine.

— JAMES BUECHLER, "JOHN SOBIESKI BURNS"

But it was running that brought Christine peace. It allowed her escape. It offered a form of freedom from the responsibilities of the everyday world. It also provided empowerment, important for a female attempting to survive in a business world with rules designed by men. The act of running created a corner from which she could not easily be pried. Christine revered the running sport for its ability to provide one hour during the workday when she could shove her business commitments aside and just run free.

— HAL HIGDON, *MARATHON: THE NOVEL*

They stood side by side, and Achilles showed them the goal. The course was set out for them from the starting-post, and the son of Oileus took the lead at once, with Ulysses as close behind him as the shuttle is to a woman's bosom when she throws the woof across the warp and holds it close up to her.

— HOMER, *THE ILIAD*

I had the road all to myeslf, and I fairly flew—leastways I had it all to myself except the solid dark, and the now-and-then glares, and the buzzing of the rain, and the thrashing of the wind, and the splitting of the thunder; and sure as you are born I did clip it along!

— MARK TWAIN, *THE ADVENTURES OF HUCKLEBERRY FINN*

Men, wives, and children stare, cry out, and run,
As it were doomsday.

— SHAKESPEARE, *JULIUS CAESAR*

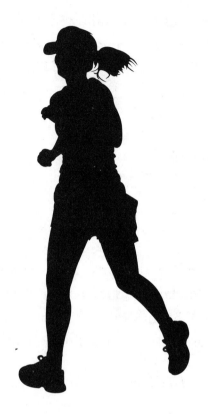

Neither have they hearts to stay,
Nor wit enough to run away.

— SAMUEL BUTLER, "HUDIBRAS"

Go, run, fly and avenge us.

— PIERRE CORNEILLE, *THE CID*

Violence upon the roads: violence of horses;
Some few have handsome riders, are garlanded
On delicate sensitive ear or tossing mane,
But wearied running round and round in their courses
All break and vanish, and evil gathers head:
Herodias' daughters have returned again.

— WILLIAM BUTLER YEATS, "NINETEEN HUNDRED AND NINETEEN"

I thought I'd run for miles, I'll bloody show him, and for awhile, maybe a quarter of an hour or so, it was a bit better, I was almost beginning to enjoy it, which he probably realized, because soon things started getting even harder; there were many more hills to climb, even a run across the grass.

— BRIAN GANVILLE, "THE OLYMPIAN"

If you had but looked big and spit at him, he'd have run.

— WILLIAM SHAKESPEARE, *THE WINTER'S TALE*

———◆———

At Marathon arrayed, to the battle shock we ran
And our mettle we displayed, foot to foot, man to man
And our name and fame shall not die.

— ARISTOPHANES, *THE ACHARNIANS*

———◆———

Like wine through clay,
Joy in his blood bursting his heart,
He died—the bliss!

— ROBERT BROWNING, "PHEIDIPPIDES"

———◆———

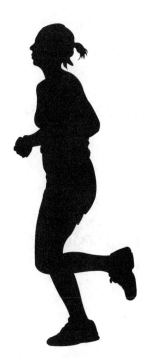

Even so close behind him was Ulysses treading in his footprints before the dust could settle here, and Ajax could feel his breath on the back of his head as he ran swiftly on.

— HOMER, *THE ILIAD*

Foley was said to offer up his running to a saint; he could offer up his too, but to some divinity that did not need to be specified: to the spirit of running perhaps.

— VICTOR PRICE, "THE OTHER KINGDOM"

But those who wait on the Lord Shall renew their strength;
They shall mount up with wings like eagles,
They shall run and not be weary
They shall walk and not faint.

— ISAIAH 40:31

On a flat road runs the well-train'd runner;
He is lean and sinewy, with muscular legs;
He is thinly clothed—he leans forward as he runs,
With lightly closed fists, and arms partially rais'd.

— WALT WHITMAN, "THE RUNNER"

Ulysses therefore carried off the mixing-bowl, for he got before Ajax and came in first.

— HOMER, *THE ILIAD*

All visible visibly
Moving things
Spin or swing,
One of the two,
Move, as the limbs
Of a runner do,
To and fro,
Forward and back,
Or, as they swiftly
Carry him
In orbit go
Round an endless track

— W. H. AUDEN, "RUNNER"

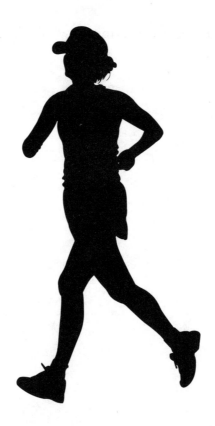

I am a feather on the bright sky
I am the blue horse that runs in the plain
I am the fish that rolls, shining, in the water

— N. Scott Momaday, "The Delight Song of Tsoai-Talee"

House Master: So, uh, how do you come to be here?

Colin Smith: [*puzzled*] I got sent, didn't I?

House Master: [*chuckles*] Yes, I know you got sent, but why?

Colin Smith: I got caught. Didn't run fast enough!

— ALAN SILLITOE, *THE LONELINESS OF THE LONG DISTANCE RUNNER*

Know ye not that they which run in a race run all, but one receiveth the prize? So run, that ye may obtain. And every man that striveth for the mastery is temperate in all things. Now they do it to obtain a corruptible crown; but we an incorruptible. I therefore so run, not as uncertainly; so fight I, not as one that beateth the air: But I keep under my body, and bring it into subjection: lest that by any means, when I have preached to others, I myself should be a castaway.

— I CORINTHIANS 9:24–27

The two men ran, pursuer and pursued,
and he who fled was noble, he behind
a greater man by far. They ran full speed,
and not for bull's hide or a ritual beast,
or any prize that men compete for; no,
but for the life of Hektor, tamer of horses.

— HOMER, *THE ILIAD*

If you can fill the unforgiving minute
With sixty second' worth of distance run
Yours is the Earth and everything that's in it
And—which is more—you'll be a Man, my son!

— RUDYARD KIPLING, "TIME"

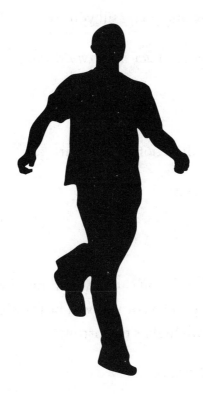

Yet that man is happy and poets sing of him who conquers with hand and swift foot and strength.

— PINDAR, GREEK POET, 500 B.C.

Begin at the beginning and go on till you come to the end; then stop.

— LEWIS CARROLL, *ALICE IN WONDERLAND*

We must travel in the direction of our fear.

— JOHN BERRYMAN

On the mountains of truth you can never climb in vain: either you will reach a point higher up today, or you will be training your powers so that you will be able to climb higher tomorrow.

— FRIEDRICH NIETZSCHE

If one advances confidently in the direction of his dreams and endeavors to live the life which he has imagined, he will meet with success unexpected in common hours.

— HENRY DAVID THOREAU

Now you will not swell the rout
Of lads that wore their honors out,
Runners whom renown outran
And the name died before the man.

— A.E. Housman

Nobody running at full speed has either a head or a body.

— William Butler Yeats

CHAPTER EIGHT

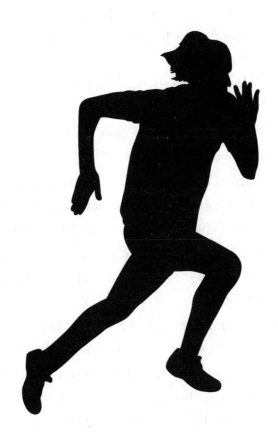

Keeping pace with the "elites"

Front Runners

The day before the Boston Marathon one year, I went for a short run on the banks of the Charles River, across the expressway, not far from the hotels where most runners stay. I was in Boston as a reporter, not as a runner, but I wanted to identify with those who would toe the starting line in Hopkinton the next day.

So I ran from my hotel to the river, a distance of about a mile. I stopped. I stretched, lying down on the grass on a warm day to do so. Then I jogged back toward my hotel at a very slow pace befitting someone whose best competitive days were well behind him.

Ahead, I spied three Kenyan runners returning to their hotel from a different direction. Using a pedestrian walkway, they crossed the expressway before I reached it. Then as we continued up a slight incline toward Boylston Street, I found that I was catching them! I could not pass. That would be an assault on reality, so I slowed and allowed the talented trio to reach the hotel before me.

Some people think that Kenyans always run fast, that every stride is at a pace near 90 percent of maximum. Not true. Like most successful elite runners, they know when to push, and they know when to rest.

The next time I saw the three Kenyans was from the press truck during the Boston Marathon. They were leading the race.

Roger Bannister

I was startled and frightened. I glanced round uneasily to see if anyone was watching. A few more steps—self-consciously . . . the earth seemed almost to move with me. I was running now, and a fresh rhythm entered my body.

— ROGER BANNISTER ON FIRST RUNNING WHEN HE WAS A CHILD

If there was a moment when things began, that was it for me.

— ROGER BANNISTER ON WATCHING ARNE ANDERSSON BEAT SYDNEY WOODERSON AT A TRACK MEET IN 1945

I'm afraid that you'll never be any good. You just haven't got the strength or build for it.

— OXFORD GROUNDSKEEPER TO ROGER BANNISTER ON RUNNING

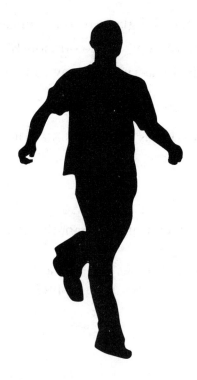

A hard-working medical student who between writing theses and delivering babies, turns his brain to the technique and theory of running.

— THE *DAILY TELEGRAPH*

We heard wonderful stories in Helsinki that Bannister would win because he had done a world-shattering time in a secret trial before leaving. MAYBE HE DID. ANYONE CAN RUN QUICKLY PAST TREES!

— THE *DAILY MIRROR* ON BANNISTER'S FAILURE AT THE HELSINKI OLYMPICS

A disaster is something which is shared between you and the public which expects something of you and which you cannot or have not fulfilled.

— ROGER BANNISTER ON THE 1952 HELSINKI OLYMPICS, WHERE HE DID NOT RUN WELL

Bannister had terrific grace, a terrific long stride, he seemed to ooze power. It was as if the Greeks had come back and brought to show you what the true Olympic runner was like.

— *DAILY MAIL* JOURNALIST TERRY O'CONNOR

Roger may tell you he has slept before a race, but he hasn't. When he goes out to run, he looks like a man going to the electric chair.

— CHRIS CHATAWAY

Stop bouncing, and you'll knock twenty seconds off.

— SECRETARY OF THE BRITISH OLYMPIC ASSOCIATION'S ADVICE TO BANNISTER WHEN HE RAN A MILE IN 4:52 IN HIS FRESHMAN YEAR AT OXFORD

[Y]ou do this because I'm the coach and I tell you.

— COACH BILL THOMAS TO BANNISTER

Does it work? Does it not? You learn by your mistakes. It's so subtle. If you run so hard that you can't recover, you haven't done any good.

— ROGER BANNISTER ON HIS TRAINING

Anyone who beats him in the Olympics at Helsinki will have to fly.

— BRITISH OFFICIAL

———◆———

Bannister has a fine, though by no means an inordinately strong physique. Many others have been as richly blessed as he. His running is a triumph of technique . . . and his success is the result of applying his intellect to the job.

— THE *DAILY TELEGRAPH*

———◆———

To say . . . "Four minutes is only a time" was presumptuous, unless I had an answer for the inevitable follow-up question—"Well, if it's possible, why don't you do it?"

— ROGER BANNISTER ON QUESTIONS FROM THE PRESS

———◆———

Nobody gets in such an emotional pitch before a race as he does.

— CHRIS CHATAWAY

———◆———

There was no longer any need for my mind to force my limbs to run faster.

— ROGER BANNISTER ON THE HEIGHT OF HIS TRAINING

———◆———

A schoolboy beat me in a quarter-mile. I could see no reason for going on.

— JOHN LANDY AFTER HE CAME BACK FROM THE BANNISTER RACE IN VANCOUVER

———◆———

It was as if all my muscles were a part of a perfectly tuned machine.

— ROGER BANNISTER ON A SUCCESSFUL RACE

———◆———

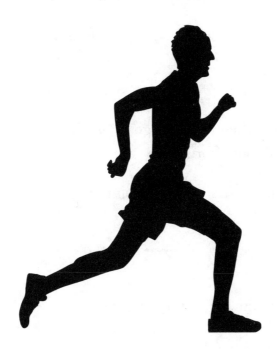

He ran like a "green" three-year-old thoroughbred having its first race in a classic—running all over the track, on the inside, then the outside, accelerating and slowing up before making his final effort, to finish fourth.

— THE *DAILY MIRROR* ON ROGER BANNISTER'S FAILURE AT THE HELSINKI OLYMPICS

By the way, I may be trying for the four-minute mile at Oxford soon.

— ROGER BANNISTER IN A LETTER TO HIS SISTER JOYCE

There comes a time when you can't go on waiting indefinitely. You just have to accept an all-out effort.

— ROGER BANNISTER TO ROGER DIMMOCK AFTER BREAKING THE FOUR-MINUTE MILE

I think I could beat him if I had the chance.

— WES SANTEE

Now life in earnest was beginning.

— ROGER BANNISTER AFTER BREAKING THE FOUR-MINUTE MILE

We honestly believed that, if you have a dream and you work to make it come true, then you really can change the world. There's just nothing you can't do.

— ROGER BANNISTER

It was the race I had to win, but I didn't.

— JOHN LANDY ON HIS LOSS AGAINST ROGER BANNISTER IN VANCOUVER

[The] art of taking more out of yourself than you've got

— ROGER BANNISTER ON RUNNING THE MILE

I will be out to win, not break records.

— ROGER BANNISTER

Roger, you only become really friendly with your opponents after you've beaten them!

— Don Macmillan to Roger Bannister

There are times the night before a race when he actually makes involuntary sounds, like a man being tortured. Roger is a hard man to comfort—if you try, he'll give you a look that goes right through you.

— Chris Chataway

Sport is about not being wrapped up in cotton wool.

— Roger Bannister

Sport is about adapting to the unexpected and being able to modify plans at the last minute.

— Roger Bannister

Sport, like all life, is about taking your chances.

— ROGER BANNISTER

——◆——

Roger hates the idea of having to beat Landy—of having thousands of people expecting him to do it. But he'll do it.

— CHRIS CHATAWAY

——◆——

What happens when a 3:59.4 miler matches strides with a 3:58 miler? It is not an academic question like the time-honored poser: What would happen if Jack Dempsey fought Joe Louis? Bannister and Landy are contemporaries, and no one will have to wait long for an answer.

— THE *NEW YORK TIMES*, AUGUST 1, 1954

——◆——

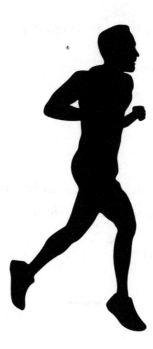

Heard a rumour that Roger ran 3:59.4, which makes a guy look rather slow!!! However, I am not unduly pessimistic.

— JOHN LANDY IN A MAY 10, 1954 LETTER TO A FRIEND

I knew you would do it one day, Roger.

> — ROGER BANNISTER'S MOTHER AFTER HE BROKE THE FOUR-MINUTE
> MILE IN 3:59.4 ON MAY 6, 1954

It is in fact only a time.

> — ROGER BANNISTER

No words could be invented for such supreme happiness.

> — ROGER BANNISTER ON BREAKING THE FOUR-MINUTE MILE

Arturo Barrios

Go knock on Arturo Barrios's door. If I was a young runner today, I'd go and hang around with the top guys like Arturo, and see what he is doing.

> — FRANK SHORTER'S ADVICE TO YOUNG RUNNERS

Josey Barthel

He had had no trainer and no compatriot with him when he came into the stadium, and he was still alone. It must have been a great solace to him on the night before the race, knowing he had nobody to disappoint.

— A. J. LIEBLING ON JOSEY BARTHEL AT THE 1952 HELSINKI OLYMPICS. BARTHEL WON THE 1,500-METER EVENT.

Dick Beardsley

It's not really bragging if you back it up.

— DICK BEARDSLEY

Holy shit, Dickie! You're leading the New York City Marathon!

— BILL SQUIRES

Dick was our sport's best-known "good guy." Everyone in the running community liked Dick.

— Bill Rodgers

———⟫•⟪———

Some of those kids come to you, they look like guppies. You wanna say, "Come on, kid, go buy some roller skates, get lost." But Dickie wasn't like that. You could tell that underneath all that aw-shucks crap he was tough as nails.

— Bill Squires

———⟫•⟪———

When I see a videotape of the race, I think of how much fun it would have been to attend as a spectator . . . just to watch. Let alone be in it. Even watching a tape today, it makes the hair on the back of my neck stand up.

— Dick Beardsley on his famous race against Alberto Salazar

———⟫•⟪———

Every marathon I ran, I knew I had a faster one in me.

— DICK BEARDSLEY

He might as well have told me I was pregnant, that's how much trouble I had believing this was happening.

— DICK BEARDSLEY ON WHEN BILL SQUIRES AGREED TO COACH HIM

We start talking workouts, and he wants to show me his training log. I said, "Jesus Christ, I don't wanna read that thing. The only thing I read is the obituaries in the morning paper to see if I'm still alive."

— BILL SQUIRES ON COACHING BEARDSLEY

Even though I'd be spent, even though I'd be cramped up, I knew with a little more training, a little more preparation, a little more experience, I could run faster.

— DICK BEARDSLEY

In 2002, the Boston Marathon brought us back for the twentieth anniversary of our race. We got to know each other. Now, among all the guys I ran with or against, Dick might be the one I feel closest to. I'll pick up the phone every few months and give him a call. I think he and I have a special bond.

— ALBERTO SALAZAR

We got into some pretty good battles. On an 8- or 10-mile run, we didn't say boo to each other for about the last five because we were trying to drive each other into the ground. The minute we'd finish, we were best friends again, but those last five miles we tried to bury each other.

— DICK BEARDSLEY ON RUNNING WITH HIS FRIEND GEORGE ROSS IN HIGH SCHOOL

It was so thick with spectators you couldn't even see how the hills went up. It was just this mass of humanity, people hanging out of trees or whatever.

— DICK BEARDSLEY ON THE BOSTON MARATHON CROWDS

Dickie had the most beautiful, efficient style I ever saw. When you watched Dickie run, violins played and little birdies flew around.

— BILL SQUIRES

Neither of us ran this well again. We didn't give an inch, and about killed each other in the process. Seriously. I was never the same again, running, mentally or physically.

— DICK BEARDSLEY ON HIS FAMOUS RACE AGAINST ALBERTO SALAZAR

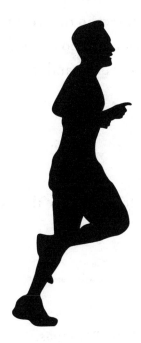

I've never been the slightest bit bored with running.

— DICK BEARDSLEY

⎯⎯◈⎯⎯

You better be careful, Dick. You're playing with fire by running so many fast marathons. The body's not designed for that kind of stress. Sooner or later you're going to have to pay a price.

— GARRY BJORKLUND

⎯⎯◈⎯⎯

I was the lead in the greatest race in the world, in front of the greatest runner in the world. It was almost too much for me to take in. And it was certainly too much for my body and mind to recover from.

— DICK BEARDSLEY

He had this fluid forefoot-striking stride that was almost effortless.

— BILL SQUIRES

After Boston, my brain told me, "No mas."

— DICK BEARDSLEY

When you push yourself to your limit, your absolute limit, and then go beyond that limit, your brain finally says, "Huh-uh, we're not going back there again. You had your shot, buddy."

— DICK BEARDSLEY

When he first came to me, I thought, "Christ, this kid must have been a beast in college; how come I never heard of him?" But when he showed me his college times, I couldn't believe how bad they were. Shit, who'd been coaching this kid, Parson Brown?

— BILL SQUIRES

Sooner or later, someone always asks about the '82 Boston. I don't mind—I like talking about it, and so does Dick. That's because we never discuss the race in terms of running a 2:08 or beating the other guy. It took us both a long, long time, but we finally realized that's not what the marathon is really about.

— ALBERTO SALAZAR

I ran the race of my life, 2:08:53. Alberto happened to run two seconds faster. All I know for certain is that I left everything I had out on that course. I didn't give an inch. Neither did Alberto. The way I look at it, there were two winners that day.

— DICK BEARDSLEY

Abebe Bikila

Abebe planted the idea that the marathon could be raced in a different way. Up until then, people would save themselves, waiting to see who would drop. He helped change the tactics.

— FRANK SHORTER

Garry Bjorklund

It's not uncommon to come across a cross-country runner; it's not uncommon to come across a track runner; and it's not uncommon to come across a road runner. But to find that mix of all three is special.

— GARRY BJORKLUND

As they prepare you to go out onto the track, you walk through a labyrinth of tunnels. You don't actually see the track until they lead you out. We sat in a room beneath the stadium, where they checked our spikes and numbers, and we could hear the pulsing of the crowds outside, reverberating. We could feel the Olympics, but not see them.

— GARRY BJORKLUND ON THE OLYMPICS

Bill Bowerman

He tailored our training to the peculiarities of our talents. When he made me take extra days of rest between workouts, I improved so much it was an epiphany.

— KENNY MOORE

Bowerman was the guide or teacher who appears in every mythic narrative at Oregon about coming of age. His main lesson was, in the words of the oracle, "Know thyself."

— KENNY MOORE

Chris Brasher

You had the feeling that he wanted to master what he was doing and literally forced himself to do it.

— A FRIEND

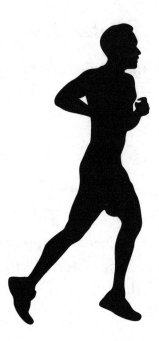

Enthusiasm was the feature you noticed about him right away. He was a thrusting sort of person.

— A FRIEND

Chris Chataway

Both were as fresh as paint at the finish.

— AAA National Coach Geoffrey Dyson after watching
Bannister and Chataway race

⎯⬧⎯

He's the one who makes me work—and keeps me amused. He will soon
run a four-minute mile himself.

— Roger Bannister

⎯⬧⎯

Eamonn Coghlan

I do love to run indoors. I love the tightness of the track. . . . The crowd
is right on top of you.

— Eamonn Coghlan

⎯⬧⎯

That magical four-minute mile barrier has set a universal standard. To run under that time is a phenomenal achievement. For the average runner, to see how close that person can come to the "almighty" gives them an indication of where they really stand.

— EAMONN COGHLAN

In certain ways, the feeling of running a mile in 3:49 is exactly the same as when I ran my first marathon in 2:25 in New York in 1991. And that sheer exhilaration that you experience is the same for a world-class runner as it is for a jogger.

— EAMONN COGHLAN

Running a fast mile feels almost like you're flying like a bird, in complete control of everything that's going on, physically and mentally. You feel absolutely fantastic, like a runaway express train that could effortlessly go on and on forever.

— EAMONN COGHLAN

I think everyone should try running a mile. People can relate to the mile.

— EAMONN COGHLAN

Bill Easton

We never run a race we don't figure we can win. If you don't feel that way, why run?

— BILL EASTON ON HIS TEAM

"Merry Christmas! . . . Be ready for hard workouts upon your return to the campus."

— BILL EASTON'S 1953 CHRISTMAS CARD TO HIS TEAM AT THE UNIVERSITY OF KANSAS

Herb Elliott

It was just another time, another progression.

— HERB ELLIOTT AFTER RUNNING A 3:54.5 MILE IN 1958

Haile Gebrselassie

Haile Gebrselassie is the best distance runner I have seen in the last quarter century, the most electrifying personality, and somewhat of an enigma, given his Ethiopian roots.

— AMBY BURFOOT

Be in no doubt Haile is the greatest distance runner the world has ever seen.

— DAVE BEDFORD

Haile is an elegant champion and a fine example of sportsmanship.

— LASSE VIREN

It makes you want to quit.

— MARK PLAATJES ON HAILE GEBRSELASSIE'S RECORD TIMES

One gold medal on in a championship is ordinary. I wanted to get two golds and be a little different.

— HAILE GEBRESELASSIE

Florence Griffith Joyner

We entered a new era with Flo-Jo on the scene, particularly for women. She was dynamic out there, very sophisticated. She put a new twist on women's competitive sports.

— USA TRACK AND FIELD PRESIDENT PATRICIA RICO

There's a very short list of instantly recognizable female athletes. Flo-Jo is one of those athletes.

— BOB WILLIAMS

She's been an inspiration for a lot of young women and men also. She has tried to give back to inner-city kids.

— 400-METER HURDLER SANDRA FARMER PATRICK

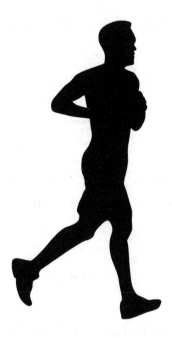

Sadly, her life has passed as rapidly as her races.

— PRIMO NEBIOLO, HEAD OF TRACK AND FIELD'S WORLD GOVERNING
BODY IAAF

Florence Griffith Joyner was one of a kind. She did many different things with style and grace.

— BERT ROSENTHAL

She just had so much style and grace and inward and outward beauty.

— SANDRA FARMER PATRICK

Florence brought a certain style to the track, something so different, with her fashionable appearance and her stunning speed.

— PATRICIA RICO

Her legacy will be one that includes kindness and interest in children and their dreams.

— BILL HYBL

It takes practice and perseverance, but as long as I hold on to my dreams, I know they'll become a reality.

— FLORENCE GRIFFITH JOYNER

Kip Keino

When Henry Rono was a young boy, Kipchoge Keino gave a talk in a stadium near Eldoret, Kenya. Rono did not go in. Instead he climbed a tree and watched the Olympian Keino talk to the crowd. Up in the tree Rono vowed he would one day be as great a runner as Keino.

— MICHAEL SANDROCK

He was a mystery. There was an aura of invincibility about him.

— FRANK SHORTER

He was a competitor in his whole lifestyle.

— MAL WHITFIELD

Sometimes I win and sometimes I don't. The cap has nothing to do with it. The race is in God's hands.

— KIP KEINO, ANSWERING REPORTERS' QUESTIONS ON WHETHER HIS ORANGE HAT HAD ANY SORT OF SIGNIFICANCE

Kipchoge was a natural. He did what he was born to do. He grew up in a good traditional society, with natural living. He didn't dissipate his energy, but stayed focused on who and what he wanted to become.

— MAL WHITFIELD

People really feared him when he was running.

— FRANK SHORTER

I think a big enemy for world-ranking African athletes like Keino is their generous nature and the readiness to run anywhere any time.

— PETER SNELL

[He ran] in his natural unfettered style, like a man running for the sheer pleasure of it.

— FRANCIS NORONHA

I gave him advice; I didn't coach him and neither did anyone else. There is a difference between philosophy and coaching. Unless you are seeing a lot of someone, spending time with them day in and day out, you are not coaching. Saying a few things is not coaching; it's giving assistance and friendship.

— MAL WHITFIELD

People sometimes say runners like my father and other Kenyan runners win because they are talented. . . . There's no secret. All there is is hard work, just training very hard. That's how my father did it, and that's how the others are doing it.

— MARTIN KEINO

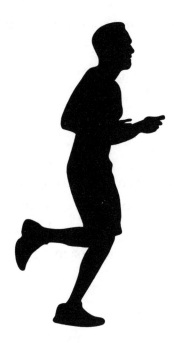

One of the athletes I admired most was Kip Keino, who was a real gentleman, highly intelligent, and a brilliant runner, so versatile. He was one of the founders of the great Kenyan distance-running history.

— ARTHUR LYDIARD

I suppose my upbringing contributed a bit to my outlook. Don't make others suffer. Try to assist them if you can.

— KIP KEINO, REFERRING TO THE BEATINGS HE RECEIVED AS A CHILD

Kip had what the best runners all have—the instinct to psych out your opponents in whatever way you can.

— FRANK SHORTER

When my father started out, he wasn't so good. He realized he could be good after he got some international exposure and was fifth in the [1964] Olympics. That's when he increased his training and that's when he got good.

— MARTIN KEINO

He wasn't cocky after he won; he was just a natural, and he was always humble.

— MAL WHITFIELD

❖

Johnny Kelley

I think the job toughened me up, climbing and walking and stooping all day. When I began my run at night, I was tired; but after a mile or so, the tiredness went away.

— THREE-TIME BOSTON MARATHON WINNER JOHNNY KELLEY ON HIS JOB AT BOSTON EDISON ELECTRIC COMPANY

❖

John Landy

While you were at the pictures, or square dancing, last Saturday night, John Landy was doing a 10-mile training run.

— HARRY HOPMAN IN THE *MELBOURNE HERALD*

I just go out there and work. I've got to punish myself to get anywhere.

— JOHN LANDY TO THE *SYDNEY MORNING HERALD*

———◆———

A certain amount of nervous energy to be released. . . . A level track with "life" in it.

— FRANK TIERNEY IN THE *SYDNEY MORNING HERALD* ON TWO OF THE CONDITIONS JOHN LANDY WOULD NEED IN ORDER TO BREAK THE FOUR-MINUTE MILE

———◆———

There is no gray—just black and white. . . . If you're hurt enough to limp, you can't run at all. If you aren't, it makes no difference.

— JOHN LANDY TO *SPORTS ILLUSTRATED*

———◆———

I'm taking no more advice from anyone. I simply want to put together the best of what I've seen.

— JOHN LANDY TO PERRY CERUTTY

At home I faced the prospect of running badly on mediocre tracks against mediocre competition in little meets attended by three people. It was too much.

— JOHN LANDY

Landy is magnificent—the greatest mile runner I have seen. On a first-class cinder track with solid opposition he'll run 3:55 for the mile.

— DENIS JOHANSSON

The only thing of which I am certain is that I have a greater capacity for punishment this season.

— JOHN LANDY

Landy has the best chance of all men today, because he is not dependent on pacemaking. He makes his own, which gives John an advantage over U.S., British and European milers.

— WES SANTEE

No one outside of sport can imagine the grind of years of continuous training. I feel I could go on for 10 years, but I don't think it's worth it.

— JOHN LANDY AFTER RUNNING A 4:02 MILE

I have always said that Landy could run 3:57.

— PERCY CERUTTY

[It gave me] equal pleasure as running 4:02 for the mile.

— JOHN LANDY ON FINDING A STENCILED HAIRSTREAK BUTTERFLY
(COLLECTING BUTTERFLIES WAS ONE OF HIS HOBBIES)

Sportsmen, as well as statesmen, carry a heavy responsibility for our good name. So long as they are of the Landy type, they will not let us down.

— *MELBOURNE AGE,* JUNE 23, 1954

I'm vicious underneath.

— JOHN LANDY

Frankly, I think the four-minute mile is beyond my capabilities. Two seconds may not sound much, but to me it's like trying to break through a brick wall.

— JOHN LANDY AFTER RUNNING A 4:02 MILE

They don't run on their toes like sprinters and paw the track with their spikes as I used to. With a higher arm carriage your knees automatically lift and you get a slightly longer stride. When it comes to the final spurt you have so much extra strength to get on your toes and sprint home.

— JOHN LANDY ON EUROPEAN RUNNERS' STYLE

He was not ebullient or over the moon. It was as if this was an entirely private achievement, something he wanted, worked for, struggled for one hell of a lot of time, and suddenly it had arrived. It was almost like having the world's press descend on your wedding night. This was entirely private to him.

— CHRIS CHATAWAY ON JOHN LANDY'S ATTITUDE AFTER HE RAN A 3:58 MILE

In any running event, you are absolutely alone. Nobody can help you.

— JOHN LANDY

[S]hort races are run without thought. In very long races you must go a great distance simply to be present in the laps that really count.

— JOHN LANDY

[A]lmost every part of the mile is important—you can never let down, never stop thinking, and you can be beaten at almost any point.

— JOHN LANDY

I suppose you could say it is like life. I had wanted to master it.

— JOHN LANDY ON RUNNING

He was all we mythologized about ourselves. Gallant, modest, idealistic, but beneath it all a champion equipped with [a] destructive will.

— SPORTSWRITER ADRIAN MCGREGOR

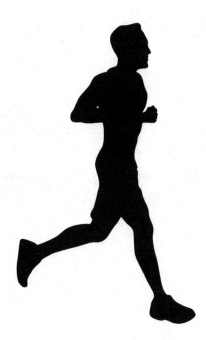

I am convinced I must have someone to grind record figures out of me. I must have someone behind me to push me out.

— John Landy

Running is not a life; I had to quit sometime. I decided that the time had come to scrub it.

— John Landy after he came back from the Bannister race in Vancouver

Running gave me discipline and self expression.

— JOHN LANDY

[Running] has all the disappointments, frustrations, lack of success and unexpected success, which all reproduce themselves in the bigger play of life.

— JOHN LANDY

Never in the history of footracing have strangers come up from nowhere to shatter or approach marks. They always bore credentials first, a background of other high-class performances. . . . [Landy] is either one of the seven wonders of the age or something's wrong somewhere.

— ARTHUR DALEY IN THE *NEW YORK TIMES*

[Running] teaches you the ability to present under pressure.

— JOHN LANDY

———◆———

[Running] teaches you the importance of being enthusiastic, dedicated, focused.

— JOHN LANDY

———◆———

Landy had tried so hard, and I am very glad that he has now succeeded. It shows that times can always be broken.

— ROGER BANNISTER AFTER LANDY BEAT HIS MILE RECORD, RUNNING A 3:58 TIME

———◆———

It was done. Finished. Next thing.

— JOHN LANDY ON HIS ATTITUDE AFTER RUNNING A 3:58 MILE

———◆———

I can do even better.

— JOHN LANDY

Carl Lewis

After I left the podium in Atlanta, I felt so fulfilled in my career that I lost my desire to compete at that level again.

— CARL LEWIS, AFTER THE ATLANTA OLYMPICS

Trust funds are not necessary anymore. They give the public a false impression that the athletes somehow are still amateur.

— CARL LEWIS

John Lodwick

It was a tremendous amount of work and a tremendous amount of fun.

> — JOHN LODWICK ON HIS YEARS AS A PROFESSIONAL RUNNER FOR NIKE'S ATHLETICS WEST TEAM

I was extremely serious about running, obviously, but I primarily thought of it as a way to know and serve God. For me, running was a way to witness.

> — JOHN LODWICK

We were young and single and caught up in something important—something that was much more than a sport.

> — JOHN LODWICK ON HIS YEARS AS A PROFESSIONAL RUNNER FOR NIKE'S ATHLETICS WEST TEAM

At times, at its best, running could even be a form of prayer.

— JOHN LODWICK

Jack Lovelock

It was all so easily accomplished, with so little outward evidence of stress and strain, as to make a four-minute mile seem just around the corner.

— *THE NEW YORK HERALD TRIBUNE* ON LOVELOCK'S 4:07.6 RACE ON JULY 15, 1933

I have now learned better than to have my races dictated by the public and the press, so I did not throw away a certain championship merely to amuse the crowd and be spectacular.

— JACK LOVELOCK, 1936 OLYMPIC GOLD MEDALIST

You mean *the* Jack Lovelock.

— ROGER BANNISTER WHEN HE MET LOVELOCK IN 1947

Billy Mills

Worry about him? I never even heard of him.

— RON CLARKE, AUSTRALIAN DISTANCE RUNNER, ON BILLY MILLS'S 10,000 VICTORY IN THE TOKYO OLYMPICS, 1964

Coming off the last turn, my thoughts changed from 'One more try, one more try, one more try. . .' to 'I can win! I can win! I can win!'

— BILLY MILLS

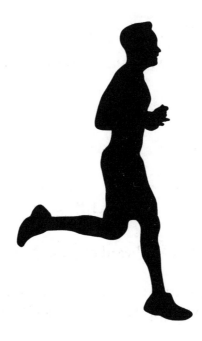

My life is a gift to me from my Creator. What I do with my life is my gift back to my Creator.

— BILLY MILLS

Paavo Nurmi

The Olympic Torch is being brought into the stadium by . . . P-A-A-V-O N-U-R-M-I.

— ANNOUNCEMENT AT THE 1952 HELSINKI OLYMPICS

———◆———

Once, it is said, he ran 40 miles from a small town to his home in Turku on the northwest coast of Finland. His wife heard a faint scratching on their back door. Thinking it was a neighborhood dog, she opened the door. There was Paavo, slumped in a heap on the doorstep, so exhausted from his run that he could not open the door.

— MICHAEL SANDROCK

———◆———

Gordon Pirie

Pirie is the most extraordinary runner the world has known, bearing in mind his amazing type of training and the distances over which he seems to be able to beat records.

— JOSEPH BINKS

Steve Prefontaine

At a very young age, he was competitive against the best in the world. He certainly wasn't scared of running against whomever.

— ALBERTO SALAZAR ON STEVE PREFONTAINE

To give anything less than your best is to sacrifice the gift.

— STEVE PREFONTAINE

His talent was not that he had great style. He didn't. It got better, I think. We worked probably harder on that than we did on anything.

— WALT MCCLURE

⬥

Pre inspired a whole generation of American distance runners to excel. He made running cool.

— ALBERTO SALAZAR

⬥

I haven't seen too many American distance men on the international scene willing to take risks. I saw some U.S. women in Barcelona willing to risk, more than men. The Kenyans risk. Steve Prefontaine risked. I risked—I went through the first half of the Tokyo race just a second off my best 5000 time.

— BILLY MILLS, GOLD MEDAL WINNER OF THE 10,000 AT THE 1964 TOKYO OLYMPICS WITH A 46-SECOND PR.

Goldarn. I wanted to run against Young more than anybody in the field. I wanted to test the veteran out. I almost said the old man, but I don't want to make him mad and give him something to use against me when we race.

> — STEVE PREFONTAINE ON RACING GEORGE YOUNG AT THE *LOS ANGELES TIMES* INDOOR MEET

He sure is a speedy little bug.

> — KERRY O'BRIEN

He had a lot of imagination and thought of all sorts of things to do out there. He worked awful hard.

> — WALT MCCLURE

The minute Pre hit the field for his jog, there was an undercurrent of enthusiasm in the crowd. It surfaced in slight cheers as he raced down the stretch. You could feel the electricity.

— GEOFF HOLLISTER

———◆———

I was really gung-ho the whole next year, 1972, trying to get into good enough shape to say, "I'm going to stick with the guy and possibly beat him in the end."

— GREG FREDERICKS

———◆———

He was self-confident, yes, sir. He wasn't cocky, as a lot of people accused him of later. He had a lot of pride, but it was constructive.

— WALT MCCLURE

———◆———

It was at the district cross country meet his sophomore year that his potential to become an outstanding runner showed itself.

— WALT MCCLURE ON STEVE PREFONTAINE

———◆———

I knew I had it in me but I had to prove it to myself. Now I'm ready to run with anybody cause I know what I can take I'll just have to polish up on my form which was not the best but not bad either.

— STEVE PREFONTAINE IN A 1969 LETTER

———◆———

Most freshmen enter college with only a vague idea of what they want to pursue as a vocation. Steve thought that he would like to major in something that would lead to a career in "insurance work or interior decorating."

— TOM JORDAN IN *PRE: THE STORY OF AMERICA'S GREATEST RUNNING LEGEND, STEVE PREFONTAINE*

———◆———

He was just pretty naïve as a freshman.

— BILL DELLINGER, PREFONTAINE'S CROSS COUNTRY COACH

———◆———

Hey, that's me, and it's pronounced Pre-fon-taine.

— STEVE PREFONTAINE WHEN A SPORTING GOODS STORE CLERK ASKED
HIM IF HE KNOW ANYTHING ABOUT A GOOD RUNNER FROM COOS BAY

———◆———

On his morning runs, I didn't check on him. I just said if you want to be
a good runner, you've got to get out there in the mornings.

— WALT MCCLURE

———◆———

As other kids who were aspiring baseball players might hear of Babe Ruth, that's how I would hear of Pre.

— ALBERTO SALAZAR

He got out on me and you get to a point where you notice, all of a sudden, that he's gotten away, and you have a complete letdown.

— GREG FREDERICKS

You can be an athlete. Athletes are very, very big in Coos Bay. You can study, try to be an intellectual, but there aren't many of those. Or you can go drag the Gut in your lowered Chevy with a switchblade in your pocket.

— STEVE PREFONTAINE ON HIS CHILDHOOD IN COOS BAY, OREGON

Pre was the hardest worker in running that I ever had by far. This is the whole thing, his intensity.

— WALT MCCLURE

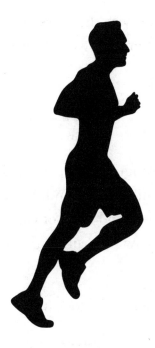

To understand Steve Prefontaine, it is necessary to know something about Coos Bay, Oregon. The town and the man find themselves similarly described: blunt, energetic, tough, aggressive.

— KENNY MOORE

Evidently, he had problems with the press or something. If you ask dumb questions, you get dumb answers, I guess.

— WALT MCCLURE

He used to run through Mingus Park, past the swimming pool and then up the steep Tenth Street hill and beyond. It's an odd thing, but although I saw him running the streets and trails of Coos Bay about a hundred times, I don't think I ever saw him running downhill. Seems like he was always going up.

— A LONGTIME RESIDENT OF COOS BAY

A couple of guys I know wave at me. Some of the bread men, garbage men, and street cleaners.

— STEVE PREFONTAINE ON HIS EARLY-MORNING RUNS IN COOS BAY

What I want is to be number one.

— STEVE PREFONTAINE

———◆———

He wouldn't take second effort—it wasn't acceptable. It was all out. When you're like that, when you start doing that, you become a lot more consistent.

— ALBERTO SALAZAR

———◆———

He was always running up and down, shouting encouragement and advice. We finally had to tell him, "Look, we'll do the coaching, you do the running."

— WALT MCCLURE

———◆———

A lady came into the store where I worked, and said, "Mrs. Prefontaine, you should go to the meets. Your son is Olympic stuff." I still remember the words.

— STEVE PREFONTAINE'S MOTHER

He was someone who didn't know any better and went out and did what he said he was going to do. We nicknamed him "The Rube."

— BILL DELLINGER

His front-running example reinforced in my mind that that was the way you showed what you were made of—lead from the front, not just wait in the back.

— ALBERTO SALAZAR

He'd like to slump over, and we'd keep hollering at him.

— WALT MCCLURE ON STEVE PREFONTAINE'S RUNNING STYLE

———◆———

Pre and Geis finished hand-in-hand and staring at each other. Not in friendship but in distrust that the other would make a last-second lunge for the tape.

— BILL DELLINGER, UNIVERSITY OF OREGON CROSS COUNTRY COACH, ON STEVE PREFONTAINE AND PAUL GEIS AT A HILITES CAMPAIGN

———◆———

[H]is talent was his control of his fatigue and his pain. His threshold was different than most of us, whether it was inborn or he developed it himself.

— WALT MCCLURE ON STEVE PREFONTAINE

———◆———

He had this magnetism that just drew people toward him. He had the personality that people would just take to. It was strange, because many times we discussed it and he said it was just the way he acted, nothing unnatural.

— RALPH MANN ON STEVE PREFONTAINE

We were against the defending state mile champion and the boy who would become the state high school cross country champion, and there was maybe a quarter mile left to go when this little guy in purple passed them and took a short lead. They just went, "Who was that?"

— WALT McCLURE

Maybe it was just his confidence, his sense of calmness.

— PAUL GEIS

I was standing on a hill. I had my binoculars, and I was probably a good half-mile or 700 yards away from the start. And I saw this guy that had the start position, but it was the look in his eyes from a half-mile distance, the intensity in his face as the gun went off. I thought, "That's got to be Pre."

— BILL DELLINGER ON FIRST SEEING STEVE PREFONTAINE

What I like most about track is the feeling I get inside after a good run.

— STEVE PREFONTAINE

Bill Rodgers

The gun goes off and the next thing I know, we pass 10 miles in 50 minutes, and there's a runner next to me—it's Bill Rodgers. It was his first race in God knows how long, and he ran 1:47 something for 20 miles. I was surprised as could be.

— AMBY BURFOOT ON A 1973 RACE

We were always moving. We'd go out and play in the woods, and I always had a lot of energy.

— BILL RODGERS ON HIS CHILDHOOD

The coach would send us off on a long run—which then might be three miles—and Bill would be far more into it than me or the other guys. I'd take off and go to my girlfriend's house, but Bill would go run for an hour.

— CHARLIE RODGERS, BILL'S BROTHER, ON HIGH SCHOOL CROSS COUNTRY DAYS

[Running] was the only area of my life where I was successful.

— BILL RODGERS

Billy was the man, and I was one of the guys who wanted to dethrone the king. It's to his credit that I had so many opportunities to try, and never did.

— GARRY BJORKLUND

When I was fired, I had time on my hands. And it was gnawing at me psychologically to do something positive with my life.

— BILL RODGERS

One of Bill's brilliant, brilliant things was that he returned every phone call from every journalist, meaning he was written up by every paper big and small.

— AMBY BURFOOT

He just toys with fields. He plays with them. It's almost a joke.

— TOMMY LEONARD

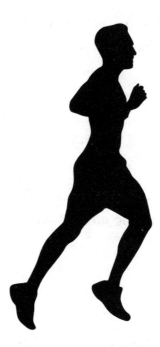

We'd go looking for butterflies, and sometimes it would get competitive, and I'd run and swoop them from under the noses of my friends.

— BILL RODGERS ON HIS CHILDHOOD

I introduced my wife to Billy, and afterwards she just couldn't believe he was the king of the roads. She thought he was just a mild-mannered schoolteacher from suburban Boston. And he was—until he laced on his shoes.

— GARRY BJORKLUND

Bill beat me like a drum. I never thought of it as personal rivalry but one from an athletic standpoint.

— FRANK SHORTER

I'm just lucky in terms of the biomechanics. I've never had a broken bone or a sprained ankle.

— BILL RODGERS

He ran with a relaxed, flowing stride, and he seemed to have the ability to go out there and hammer people in the middle of the race and not leave it to the end.

— AMBY BURFOOT

———◆———

Billy was very capable of banging with anyone. He always respected the competition; he respected the other runners and saw everyone he was racing against as being capable of beating him. He was always friendly to his competition after races, never aloof.

— CHARLIE RODGERS

———◆———

Billy was a little intimidating when he was racing. He was a nice guy, except when he was racing. In a race, he became an animal and would do anything to beat you.

— BENJI DURDEN

———◆———

Bill was very gifted, and was unusual in that he's probably gotten the fastest marathon times off the slowest track times of anyone. It was incredible, and I was always fascinated by that.

— FRANK SHORTER

I've had a streak, and I'm into my prime years, but it ain't going to last forever.

— BILL RODGERS IN 1979

Billy was "the man" when I was growing up in Massachusetts. Anyone who has ever met Billy knows he's a real nice guy, and always helpful for younger runners.

— MARK COOGAN

It was his relaxation that most amazed me. He seemed to be able to run with almost complete detachment from the mental and physical effort involved.

— AMBY BURFOOT

———◆———

[Boston was] Bill's town, its people his supporters, its streets, from Commonwealth Avenue to the suburbs, his playground.

— JOURNALIST ON BILL RODGERS AT THE 1978 BOSTON MARATHON

———◆———

Oh, oh. There are 10 miles to go and number one, my stomach hurts; number two, Bjorklund looks good out there; and number three, here is Seko, whose presence reminds me of my loss to him in Fukuoka.

— BILL RODGERS ON THE 1978 BOSTON MARATHON IN HIS BOOK *THE RUNNER*

———◆———

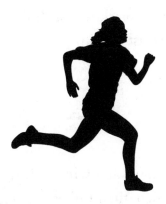

It was fun for him while for the rest of us, it was a lot of hard work. We'd be croaking out there, and Bill would go out and do more. He loved it.

— CHARLIE RODGERS ON HIGH SCHOOL CROSS COUNTRY DAYS

I was scared of someone coming up on me. . . . I didn't want it taken away. I could taste the third win.

— BILL RODGERS ON WINNING THE 1978 BOSTON MARATHON

In his day, you could throw a brick wall at Billy and he'd come through it and wouldn't even have dust on him.

— GARRY BJORKLUND

It was a nasty day, raining hard and windy. Billy caught up to me, looked over, and surged. I responded, then Billy surged again, and I responded again. This went on for three miles. Finally, he looked over at me and growled. Just growled, "Arrghhh!" and put on another surge, getting away from me with a mile to go. It had just pissed him off that I made him work so hard.

— BENJI DURDEN

All Bill ever wanted was a medal. He wasn't greedy. It didn't matter what color it was: gold, silver, or bronze. As long as it was a medal, even a bronze, it would have been enough. People don't understand that the only thing Billy doesn't have is a medal.

— BOB SEVENE

I don't think there's another road runner in the country who does the promotional work I do, who has the schedule I have. In fact, one of my greatest dreams is to get Rod Dixon and Herb Lindsay and a few others out there doing everything I do, on my schedule, and then we'd be even.

— BILL RODGERS IN 1982

Every time he beat me I became more resolved. I would test him and could never find a flaw. He was a real, real student of the sport.

— GARRY BJORKLUND

You can't burn the candle all the time. If you put in long miles as a teenager, how are you going to do it for twenty years after that?

— BILL RODGERS

He never got hurt; the guy's amazing that way. He was very bright in his training. He didn't train too much, and he didn't train too little.

— BOB SEVENE

I always thought of myself as a marathoner.

— BILL RODGERS

❖

What struck me most about Bill was that he would stop at every corner bakery and buy the gooiest pastries he could find, the kind with green frosting on them. He could eat *anything*.

— PABLO VIGIL ON BILL RODGERS

❖

Obviously, he had something different in his mind to train the way he did. He had the ability to push himself as hard as anyone.

— CHARLIE RODGERS

❖

We didn't begrudge Billy [his prize money]. It's hard to begrudge Billy.

— BENJI DURDEN

❖

My advice to young runners is to concentrate on track and cross-country. Take the gradual approach. Then, when you are in your twenties, experiment with longer road races. Just take a low-key approach. You can't tell in one year or two years what you are going to do.

— BILL RODGERS

He was dedicated and persevered, and was very smart about things. He had the sense not to go overboard in his training.

— CHARLIE RODGERS

[T]heir personalities still carry importance at races even now.

— BOB SEVENE ON BILL RODGERS AND FRANK SHORTER

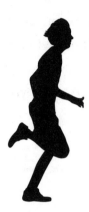

It's still fun. In some ways it's still exactly the same as it was the first day I went out for cross-country, although I don't think people believe me when I say that. But it's true. It's just like the beginning. I just love to run.

— BILL RODGERS

[As a *Sports Illustrated* writer] I cared more about evocative detail, about the image of an opal-pale Rodgers, caught at 4:00 A.M. in the refrigerator's light after a 30-mile day, eating mayonnaise with a tablespoon from the jar, asking with perfect quizzicality, "Do I run so much to eat like this, or do I eat like this to run so much?"

— KENNY MOORE

I don't feel quite so smooth when I'm running now, like I'm always running uphill or against a headwind. But I get inspired by progress, which is why I like running. You can always improve through your efforts.

— BILL RODGERS IN 1996

Alberto Salazar

If there are no injuries or unforeseen developments . . . well, the facts are plain; I'm the fastest man in the race.

— ALBERTO SALAZAR BEFORE THE 1982 BOSTON MARATHON

I always claim that the marathon is just another race to me. But Billy [Bill Rodgers] insists that someday the marathon could humble you.

— ALBERTO SALAZAR

After Boston, I was never quite the same. I had a few good races, but everything became difficult. Workouts that I used to fly through became an ordeal. And eventually, of course, I got so sick that I wondered if I'd ever get well.

— ALBERTO SALAZAR

Alberto was a mess by comparison [to Dick Beardsley]. But it didn't matter because Alberto was such a tiger, he could stand so much pain.

— BILL SQUIRES

You could say that I choked at the Olympics, but I never quit. I don't quit. I'm not going to quit. If you quit and drop out, you're always going to have that moment of doubt.

— ALBERTO SALAZAR ON THE 1984 LOS ANGELES OLYMPICS

I made a vow never to quit in a race, even if I had to walk in.

— ALBERTO SALAZAR

———⬥———

There hasn't been a Boston Marathon since where the two favorites ran together all the way from Hopkinton, doing everything possible to beat each other, neither one giving an inch. I think it was the greatest American distance race.

— ALBERTO SALAZAR ON THE 1982 BOSTON MARATHON

———⬥———

When people say I can't do something, it just makes me doubly determined.

— ALBERTO SALAZAR

———⬥———

You can always look back and say, well, if I had done this or that differently, maybe things would have been different. But in my case, I think I was as smart as I could be at the time. At times I may have overtrained, but I truly don't believe my career was ended by overtraining.

— ALBERTO SALAZAR

For much of the last 10 years, I hated running. I hated it with a passion. I used to wish for a cataclysmic injury in which I would lose one of my legs. I know that sounds terrible, but if I had lost a leg, then I wouldn't have to torture myself anymore.

— ALBERTO SALAZAR TO A REPORTER IN 1994

It made my win all the sweeter, to prove my critics wrong.

— ALBERTO SALAZAR

I did what I aimed to do in that race. That's the best you can expect out of life. Everything went perfectly during that run. It was a once-in-a-lifetime experience.

— ALBERTO SALAZAR ON WINNING THE NEW YORK CITY MARATHON
AND SETTING A WORLD RECORD

Most of the pressure I ever felt was self-imposed. I put a lot of pressure on myself. More than I should have, more than was healthy.

— ALBERTO SALAZAR

I think it comes down to pride in the end. Not proud, necessarily, that you're better than everybody else, but that you are tougher than anybody else. That if you lose, you are going to make whomever you are running against pay.

— ALBERTO SALAZAR

Al, I can't thank you enough for pushing me all the way up to the end.

— DICK BEARDSLEY

———◆◆◆———

When I didn't run well, I didn't throw tantrums, but inside I was very mad at myself. I would be hard on myself for weeks or even months afterwards.

— ALBERTO SALAZAR

———◆◆◆———

When a marathon was over, it was like a huge weight had lifted off my shoulders. I think that the best moment of a marathon was just afterward, soaking in the tub, with no more people around, no more expectations.

— ALBERTO SALAZAR

———◆◆◆———

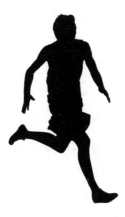

I look at that marathon as the epitome of what running is all about.

— ALBERTO SALAZAR ON THE 1982 BOSTON MARATHON

⟫◆⟪

Joan Benoit Samuelson

All athletes who strive for excellence share the same story.

— JOAN BENOIT SAMUELSON

⟫◆⟪

I run. I am a runner. I am an athlete.

— JOAN BENOIT SAMUELSON

———◆———

In March, 1983, the Friday before the World Cross-Country Championships in Gateshead, England, Benoit took me on a 10-mile run. She picked it up until I was using everything I had to stay with her. Then, up a long English hill in the rain, she became the first woman ever to run away from me.

— KENNY MOORE

———◆———

Women's running has come of age, thanks in great measure to the incomparable strides of Joan Samuelson.

— KATHRINE SWITZER

———◆———

Joan is a world-class athlete in touch with the most important aspects of physical endurance and perseverance and of striving to realize a dream despite any obstacles.

— GLORIA AVERBUCH

No athlete was ever tougher than Joan Benoit, and no one more defining in her cycle of injury, recovery, victory, and injury—of love and loving too much.

— KENNY MOORE ON JOAN BENOIT SAMUELSON

———————

Even as Benoit won the first women's Olympic marathon in 1984, I knew she was a legend. . . . I tried to see such rare creatures as exemplars of the humanly possible, templates for the generations.

— KENNY MOORE

———————

I don't have the stereotypical tall and lean runner's physique. In fact, I sometimes think people look at me and wonder how I've become an elite runner.

— JOAN BENOIT SAMUELSON

———————

Wes Santee

Guys like that never get whipped in their minds. Even when they get beat, they're not beat.

— DON HUMPHREYS

I just don't like to fiddle around. If I was told to get the hoe, I'd run to get it. If I had to go to the barn, I'd run.

— WES SANTEE ON HIS CHILDHOOD ON A RANCH

Santee's not human.

— GEORGETOWN COACH

I didn't think it was so fast.

— WES SANTEE TO A REPORTER AFTER HE RAN A MILE IN 4:02.4, AN AMERICAN RECORD

Santee struck out above every other athlete like the Aleutian Islands into the Bering Sea.

— *DES MOINES REGISTER*

I don't know when it will be, but I'll run it, you can be sure of that. I'm as certain I can run the four-minute mile as you are that you can drive your car home.

— WES SANTEE TO A JOURNALIST

Santee is the greatest prospect for the four-minute mile America has yet produced. He not only has the physical qualifications, but the mental and spiritual as well.

— DRAKE UNIVERSITY COACH

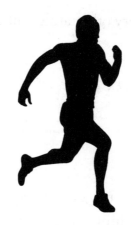

I just want to make the Olympic team. Time or race isn't important.

— WES SANTEE IN 1952

<hr/>

The guy has a lot of poise, a lot of self-assurance. He'll tell you what he can do, and you think maybe he's bragging a little, and then he goes right ahead and does it.

— A SPECTATOR

I don't want to run with you guys, none of you want to do better. You're all just out there running.

— WES SANTEE TO HIS TEAM, THE JAYHAWKS, IN 1953

You're the one to run the four-minute mile. But you still need to improve. You're going to have to do different workouts than everybody else. You need to put more pressure on yourself.

— BILL EASTON TO WES SANTEE

When I'm going to give a speech, like to young Marines, I will plan my whole day around that so I am mentally and physically alert. You can't separate these when you're performing, same as if I was running an event. I still eat my toast, tea, and honey.

— WES SANTEE

For me to drive myself. . . . I could do it up to a point, but there was something about competition that raised the bar.

— WES SANTEE ON COMPETITION

Some night Santee's going to travel around that course like the wind and then he'll not only run the four-minute mile but he'll cut three or four seconds off that goal.

— EDGAR HAYES

I am confident that I can beat any and all comers in a mile footrace.

— WES SANTEE

You remember the old story about how Babe Ruth took two strikes and then pointed to the spot where he was going to sock a home run on the next pitch? And you remember the Babe went ahead and did it? Well, that's the way Santee is.

— A SPECTATOR

I just can't talk. There's no use trying to be objective, because I can't. I get all tied in knots.

— WES SANTEE'S FIANCÉE ON WATCHING HER HUSBAND-TO-BE RACE

————◆————

There still is the challenge to see who will be the first American to break the four-minute mile. The time is still not as low as it can be run.

— WES SANTEE

————◆————

Wes Santee isn't going to let a little old thing like matrimony disrupt his plans for fast running.

— THE *KANSAS CITY STAR*

————◆————

Pay by Check. It will travel as swiftly and as tirelessly as our great miler!

— AN ADVERTISEMENT FROM THE STOCKGROWERS STATE BANK

Having to compete for the university, I've had to run everything from soup to nuts. I haven't had time to concentrate.

— WES SANTEE

Ⓐ

That means Landy and Wes Santee can never break the four-minute mile first.

— CHRIS BRASHER

Ⓐ

I am not exceptionally disappointed. Of the milers capable of doing it, Bannister is the one I'd just as soon have seen break it.

— WES SANTEE

Ⓐ

You still have more running to do.

— BILL EASTON TO WES SANTEE

Ⓐ

If you hooked Bannister onto the Twentieth Century Limited, he couldn't beat Santee.

— WES SANTEE

I'm going to train as hard as I can and sacrifice everything I have to bring the mile record back to the United States.

— WES SANTEE

The process of running a lot of miles between 4:04 and 4:06 will put Wes in the proper mental state for his major efforts outdoors. A great miler has to feel himself capable of cutting two or three seconds off his time, should the necessity arise.

— BILL EASTON

Hard work pays off. You have to be just as disciplined to run a business as you do to train for an athletic event.

— WES SANTEE

It's like someone pulls you along. I loved to be behind. . . . I judge my pace against his pace, and I'm coming on him. When I catch up and pass, it's great.

— WES SANTEE ON COMPETITION

Frank Shorter

Many people feel that Frank, simply because he won the gold medal in 1972, is inevitably number 1. No matter what I or any other marathoner has done since 1972, Frank is number 1.

— BILL RODGERS

You're really Frank Shorter, eh? . . . . What happened to you at Montreal?

— A CHARLESTON CAB DRIVER UPON LEARNING HE WAS DRIVING SHORTER, WHO WON OLYMPIC GOLD IN MUNICH IN 1972 AND SILVER IN MONTREAL IN 1976.

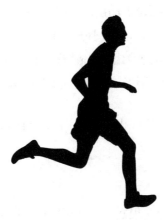

[I learned] how suddenly aggressive I could become, not unlike the aggression all runners suddenly feel when their concentration and peace of mind are broken by a threatening dog or motorist.

— FRANK SHORTER ON THE 1973 MAINICHI MARATHON IN JAPAN, WHERE A PHOTOGRAPHER TOOK A PICTURE OF HIM WHILE HE WAS STOPPING TO PEE

———◆———

What Bill and Frank did was promote running, and it boomed.

— JACK McDONALD

———◆———

Billy said, "I'm going to take Frank out." He was on a vendetta. It was nothing against Frank personally, but rather what Frank represented as the best runner in the world. Billy had full intention of being the best in the world, and he knew he'd have to beat Frank to do that.

— BOB SEVENE ON BILL RODGERS AND SHORTER

Frank Shorter looks like he always looks, not haggard, up on his toes.

— ERICH SEGAL ON SHORTER AT THE 1972 MUNICH OLYMPICS

If your reaction in the Olympics is such that you even think about whether you're going to go, it's too late.

— FRANK SHORTER

Frank had a rational judgment of what he could do. If he had a cold, or was busy in law school, he was always able to make a judgment not to kill himself and stay healthy.

— KENNY MOORE

That's not Frank! That's not Frank. It's an imposter! Get that guy off the track! How can this happen in the Olympic Games? It's bush league; get rid of that guy; there is Frank Shorter; that's Frank; come on, Frank, you won it. I wonder what Frank Shorter is thinking.

— ABC COMMENTATOR ERICH SEGAL AT THE 1972 MUNICH OLYMPICS, WHEN A YOUNG GERMAN PRETENDING TO BE SHORTER RAN ONTO THE TRACK

Part of the ability to win big races is that you truly are thinking only up to the finish line, and not worried about what's going to happen.

— FRANK SHORTER

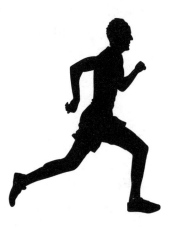

When we were business rivals [for sportswear companies], we were not as friendly, perhaps, and I said some negative things I sort of regret now.

— BILL RODGERS

What I notice about the Olympics now, part of the human interest aspect of it, implied or overt, is the kind of loss of future income that comes from a failure or for not winning. It's so apparent now. . . . [A]t Munich, that was not how the Olympics were viewed. The goal was to be the best in the world on that particular day.

— FRANK SHORTER

What really separated Frank from the other runners was his mental edge, in workouts and in races.

— PABLO VIGIL

———⊰•⊱———

I've never heard Frank say he hated someone, and he never got up by putting someone else down. He was always excellent at analyzing what he was good at and what his opponents were good at, and he'd devise a training program to help him beat them.

— LOUISE SHORTER

———⊰•⊱———

No one in the world is training as hard as we are right now.

— FRANK SHORTER TO STEVE PREFONTAINE WHEN THEY RAN 10 MILES DURING A BLIZZARD IN TAOS, COLORADO

———⊰•⊱———

He always knew how to run within himself.

— KENNY MOORE

———⊰◈⊱———

I've always been flattered that Jack Foster, in his book, said I was the only person he never really thought he could beat. I took that as the ultimate compliment from a peer, whether it was true or not.

— FRANK SHORTER

———⊰◈⊱———

When you are really successful you have an aura about you that makes opponents not only a little bit wary of you, but makes them a little bit afraid of you, and consider you a threat.

— FRANK SHORTER

———⊰◈⊱———

This unknown and unchosen star of the event turned out to be personable, articulate, penetratingly intelligent about running, and not about to be shoved into any standard media-jock package.

> — JOHN JEROME ON SHORTER'S PERFORMANCE AT THE MUNICH MARATHON IN 1972

You may run that fast again, but then again, you may not.

> — RON HILL TO FRANK SHORTER

My strategy was to incorporate track-racing strategy into what had before been more a race of attrition.

> — FRANK SHORTER

I can stand abuse better than just about anybody.

> — FRANK SHORTER

I have probably run through more airports than anyone in the country.

— FRANK SHORTER

———◆———

There's still a little starstruck voice inside me that says "Frank Shorter!" every time I see him

— JOAN BENOIT SAMUELSON

———◆———

Probably if I hadn't been injured, none of these businesses would have worked out as well, and I wouldn't be doing TV at all. But looking back, if I'd had the choice, I'd rather have been able to run.

— FRANK SHORTER ON HIS NEW CAREER AFTER HIS ANKLE INJURIES

———◆———

If a television producer isn't reading about road racing and track and field and feeling it is a hot item, he will not make an effort to put it on television.

— FRANK SHORTER ON THE IMPORTANCE OF PROMOTING RUNNING IN THE UNITED STATES

I know I'm training well when I get the right injuries.

— FRANK SHORTER

You can create all the equivalents you want, but I'll tell you what— nothing beats winning.

— FRANK SHORTER

They are different personalities, but each wanted to be the best he possibly could be and beat the other guy.

— AMBY BURFOOT ON BILL RODGERS AND FRANK SHORTER

The ability to recover goes away as you age. What I've found is that my recovery is slower, and I can't do the pounding.

— FRANK SHORTER

Together, [Bill Rodgers and Frank Shorter] inspired America in its great running boom. And having done that, they seemed tinged by faint embarrassment. Perhaps they just didn't want it to look like they had *ordered* everyone into the streets.

— KENNY MOORE

It's how you act, what you do, the personality you establish so you have the opposition more worried about what you are doing than about what they are doing.

— FRANK SHORTER

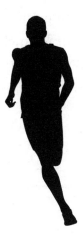

We were two individuals who both wanted to be the best in the U.S., and being the best in the U.S. at that time pretty much meant you were the best in the world.

— FRANK SHORTER ON HIMSELF AND BILL RODGERS

There was something about all those miles, all those minutes of TV coverage through the streets of Munich, something about that silken, light-footed stride and flying hair that lodged forever in our consciousness. Running. Somehow it looked . . . glorious.

— JOHN JEROME ON SHORTER'S PERFORMANCE AT THE MUNICH
  MARATHON IN 1972

———◆———

Franz Stampfl

In a way, I knew that he didn't know any better than I did whether or not I would win, because it was a total unknown quantity, but just hearing someone say the things—by then I knew what he would say—was useful.

— CHRIS CHATAWAY

———◆———

Fear is the strongest driving-force in competition. Not fear of one's opponent, but of the skill and high standard which he represents; fear, too, of not acquitting oneself well. In the achievement of greater performances, of beating formidable rivals, the athlete defeats fear and conquers himself.

— FRANZ STAMPFL

He invested with magic this whole painful business of trying to run fast. He made you feel that this would be the most wonderful thing. It would put you along with Michelangelo, Leonardo da Vinci, if you could do it, and he was quite convinced you *could* do it.

— CHRIS CHATAWAY

Pekka Vasala

It is suicidal for other runners to copy my hill sessions without adequate background.

> — PEKKA VASALA, FINNISH MIDDLE DISTANCE RUNNER WHO OUTKICKED KIP KEINO AT MUNICH OLYMPICS IN 1972 WINNING THE 1500 METERS IN 3:36.3

I didn't mind getting second. He's the best in the world.

> — STEVE PREFONTAINE

Lasse Viren

[H]e could win at his will, whenever he decided to go. Everyone just hung around and waited for him to go.

> — FRANK SHORTER

He put his elbows on his knees and just slowly looked around at everyone in the room, one by one, as if to say, "I'm here, guys." And the race was over then. I've never seen a presence like that.

— GARRY BJORKLUND ON VIREN BEFORE THE 1976 MONTREAL OLYMPICS

He had a very smooth stride that essentially did not change as he accelerated in the final laps.

— FRANK SHORTER

It was like the best chess match you'll ever see. They were outmatched mentally as well as physically.

— EINO ROMPPANEN ON VIREN AND HIS OPPOSITION AT THE 1976 MONTREAL OLYMPICS

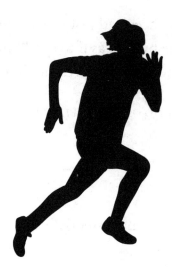

Lasse did exactly what you are supposed to do. However he did it, he created the ability to race in a way that other people felt they could not duplicate.

— FRANK SHORTER

❖

[He has] a tremendous strength of character, which is such that even if he finishes last in a race that is not important, then he genuinely does not worry.

— BRENDAN FOSTER

[E]verybody has beaten Lasse at one time or another. But nobody beats him at the Olympics.

— FRANK SHORTER

In Finland, we have a saying, "Big words don't fell the trees." That's what Lasse did in his running. His races speak louder than his words.

— EINO ROMPPANEN

Race director Scott Keenan used to say, "Foot races are like horse races; you can either assemble an exciting field, or bring in the Secretariat." That's what Lasse Viren was: a Secretariat.

— GARRY BJORKLUND

An athlete's career is a brief lightning flash; let me do as much as I can with it before it ends.

— LASSE VIREN

Unlike most distance runners, he did not switch to a sprinter's gait in a furious drive to the finish. Somehow he was able to maintain his form . . . and simply run faster.

— FRANK SHORTER

Lasse was the most talented runner ever.

— RODOLFO GOMEZ

When you look at why Lasse became Lasse, you have to look at the history, the heritage, and the culture of Finland. From the time they are kids, Finnish youth are ingrained with the idea that Finns are great athletes, and so we have that mentality. There is something Finns have that makes them think they can overcome incredible odds.

— Eino Romppanen

It looked like he was out for a Sunday stroll. There was absolutely no doubt in anybody's mind about what was going to happen.

— Garry Bjorklund on Viren at the 1976 Montreal Olympics

The man was ready, all right. I told myself, "The only thing you can do is stay as close to him as possible, because he's going to win."

— Frank Shorter on competing against Viren

Sisu is guts, and you know when someone has it. And Lasse had it.

— EINO ROMPPANEN ON VIREN AND THE FINNISH TERM *SISU*

Priscilla Welch

Before my marathon in London [in 1981], [Dave] told me I could run three hours, and I ran 2:59. I had to walk near the end, and I was thinking, "Dave said I could do three hours," and so I believed I could.

— PRISCILLA WELCH ON HER HUSBAND

I saw my times improving, and the more I did well, the more I wanted to see what was over the next ridge.

— PRISCILLA WELCH

I was very conscious of how old I was, and that there was so much to do before time ran out. It was like an exciting game.

— PRISCILLA WELCH ON BECOMING A RUNNER

I didn't start out wanting to be an international athlete, but the more I did the better I got.

— PRISCILLA WELCH

Dave saw in Cilla not just the characteristics of a great runner, but also a talent that was far from developed. With a patient, disciplined, but extensive program over time, Dave was able to turn her into one of the foremost marathoners of her time.

— PAUL CHRISTMAN ON DAVE AND PRISCILLA WELCH

We were running innocent until then. There was nothing planned before that, just put your head down and go. I was just running for the enjoyment of running. After that, we tried to put the icing on the cake.

— PRISCILLA WELCH ON WHAT CHANGED AFTER SHE FINISHED THIRD IN THE NEW YORK CITY MARATHON IN 1983

It was a case of loving what I was doing and the challenge of it.

— PRISCILLA WELCH

Priscilla never let chronological age be a barrier. She took a chance in New York and it worked.

— PAUL CHRISTMAN

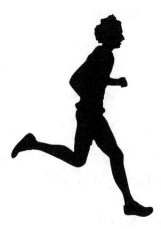

I think there must be a little bit of talent there, but talent doesn't take you a long way. I'm lucky I found something I liked to do.

— PRISCILLA WELCH

[My thoughts about moving to the United States were], we'll come to the States and experience road running here. If we're broke, we'll go back and sweep the roads. We were prepared to take the gamble.

— PRISCILLA WELCH

If you like it, pursue it.

— PRISCILLA WELCH

I don't think 40, and I certainly don't feel 40. I don't even think 40 is old. It's only early middle age. I think 80 is old.

— PRISCILLA WELCH IN 1984

The men seemed to be having a lot more fun than me. They were waving at the cameras. I had blinders on. I was totally focused on my race.

— PRISCILLA WELCH ON THE 1987 NEW YORK CITY MARATHON, WHICH SHE WON

If you want to keep putting in the performances you were putting in when you were in your early twenties, you'll notice a difference if you're eating junk. And these runners wonder why their performances have gone bad.

— PRISCILLA WELCH

Keeping the immune system healthy and the body chemically balanced while running is so important. Resting isn't poppycock. It's for real. Otherwise, your immune system gets out of whack. The defending forces get confused and *bam!* you have something serious on your hands.

— PRISCILLA WELCH

I look at my disease as a friend to me. It forced me to take a proper rest, after ten or eleven years at the top. I had to have the disease in order to stop.

— PRISCILLA WELCH ON HER BREAST CANCER

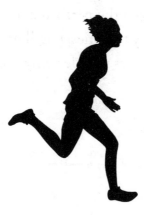

I wasn't ever afraid of the cancer, but I was annoyed. It was an interruption, because I was turning 48 and time was getting on for my running. But I heeded the message. And now that I've come out the other end, I can help other ladies go through the same thing.

— PRISCILLA WELCH ON HER BREAST CANCER

[N]ow I'm focusing on masters, whereas before it was the open. It's getting a lot harder because there's a lot of little jackrabbits in there. The masters division is getting more and more interesting.

— PRISCILLA WELCH

I may want to take up another challenge, use my brains and not my feet. Heaven forbid my brain starts working!

— PRISCILLA WELCH

———◆———

[I]t's harder to recover from an injury, and it's twice as hard mentally as well.

— PRISCILLA WELCH ON GETTING OLDER

———◆———

You don't even have to run; just do something to keep the body healthy, keep the mind healthy. That way if something does come along, you're able to cope with it.

— PRISCILLA WELCH'S ADVICE TO BREAST CANCER PATIENTS

———◆———

Cilla told me after the race that she reckoned she could take an hour off that time. She didn't realize that if she did, it would be a world record.

> — DAVE WELCH, PRISCILLA WELCH'S HUSBAND, ON PRISCILLA'S FIRST MARATHON, THE STOCKHOLM MARATHON, IN WHICH SHE RAN A 3:26 AND CAME IN NINTH

Running was exciting, and the more I ran the better I got. It was a fun time, and all so new.

> — PRISCILLA WELCH

Grete Waitz

If anyone had to choose a queen of the road, it would be Grete Waitz.

> — FRED LEBOW

Before the race I wasn't nervous. I felt great.

— GRETE WAITZ BEFORE HER FIRST NEW YORK CITY MARATHON

The night before the race, we treated ourselves to a nice restaurant complete with a four-course meal of shrimp cocktail, baked potato, red wine, and ice cream.

— GRETE WAITZ ON THE NIGHT BEFORE HER FIRST NEW YORK CITY MARATHON, IN 1978

By mile nineteen. . . . I stopped feeling so great. I knew my body had reached unknown territory, never having run so far.

— GRETE WAITZ ON HER FIRST TIME RUNNING THE NEW YORK CITY MARATHON, IN 1978

My biggest problem was not being able to convert the miles to meters, my measurement system. And since I didn't speak English that well, I was too embarrassed to ask where the heck I was.

— GRETE WAITZ

My quads were beginning to cramp so I decided to try and drink water, but I had never experienced this quick form of drinking before and kept spilling the water all over myself. It is definitely an acquired skill, something to be practiced beforehand.

— GRETE WAITZ

I continued running strong, but having no idea what mile I was on or where this place called Central Park was, I began to get annoyed and frustrated. Every time I saw a patch of trees, I thought, "Oh, this must be Central Park," but no.

— GRETE WAITZ

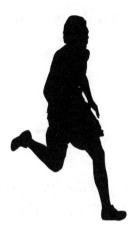

It was easy for about eighteen miles, then I really felt the difference between a marathon and the other things I had been doing.

— GRETE WAITZ ON HER FIRST NEW YORK CITY MARATHON

Never, ever am I going to do this again!

— GRETE WAITZ AFTER HER FIRST OF NINE NEW YORK CITY MARATHONS

Emil Zatopek

Emil is truly the originator of modern intensive training.

> — FRED WILT

Yes, maybe I was not the favorite for 10,000 meters, because there was world-record holder Viljo Heino of Finland. But he was used to practicing near the Arctic Circle, and in London it was a tropical gale, and Heino was unhappy with this climate.

> — EMIL ZATOPEK ON RACING VILJO HEINO AT THE 1948 LONDON OLYMPICS

He thoroughly deserved his success because he is the hardest trained athlete in the world.

> — JOHN LANDY ON EMIL ZATOPEK AND HIS THREE OLYMPIC GOLD MEDALS

I understood after the sixth kilometer that I was strong, because [the commentator] says, "After six kilometers, Zatopek is running in better time than Viljo Heino for world record." Oh, really? And the young people yell, "We want world record." And I started to run, and I ran world record.

— EMIL ZATOPEK ON A RACE IN 1949

While he goes for a twenty-mile training run on his only free day, we lie here panting with exhaustion, moaning that the gods are unkind to us, and that we're too intelligent to train hard.

— CHRIS CHATAWAY ON EMIL ZATOPEK

Zatopek had no fear of becoming "burned out."

— FRED WILT

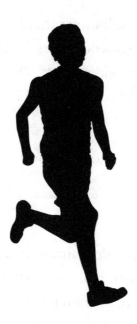

No, no, no, no. I was not very talented. My basic speed was low. Only with willpower, eee, ahhhh, was I able to reach this world best standard in long-distance running.

— EMIL ZATOPEK

We should have thrown him out angrily, and blamed our failure the following day on his disturbing our non-existent sleep. But Zatopek gave him a twenty-minute interview. Then when he found the reporter hadn't a bed for the night, he offered him half his own.

— ROGER BANNISTER RECALLING THE NIGHT BEFORE THE 1952
HELSINKI OLYMPICS, WHEN A REPORTER INTERRUPTED THEM

One thing people forget about Emil is that at any meet, such as the Olympics, he was the focal point for all the other runners. Emil could be in a room, in the middle of Swedes, Englishmen, Germans, Russians, Hungarians, Czechoslovakians, and all conversation bounced off of him, because he was a linguist. Russians and Americans would be talking, with Emil doing the translating.

— JOHN DIXLER

Finland is wonderful for the long-distance runner.

— EMIL ZATOPEK

[Emil Zatopek's training philosophy] was to work as hard as possible so that a race seemed comparatively easy. He felt that strength and energy only increase through continual testing.

— FRED WILT

———◆◆———

Four hundred meters to sprint. For me, it was very easy . . . to sprint 400 meters for most runners, it is very difficult, because maybe if you try, you will be in 200 meters full of fatigue.

— EMIL ZATOPEK

———◆◆———

Zatopek isn't human in his achievement, yet he's as intelligent as any other athlete running.

— CHRIS CHATAWAY

———◆◆———

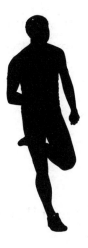

With all their energy, everybody tries to do their best. This struggle, it stays very deep in your mind. And it produces great respect among adversaries. It is this quality I esteem, not only by winning to get congratulations, but also by losing.

— EMIL ZATOPEK ON FRIENDSHIPS IN ATHLETICS

Zatopek's '52 Olympics rates as one of the greatest performances in history, and it's unlikely to ever be duplicated. To do that well in three events in the Olympics was as much a mental domination as a physical one. It was one of the greatest examples of combining psychological and physical tactics.

— FRANK SHORTER

I was able to change this quantity of training into quality of running. But nowadays, it is not good to recommend young sportsmen to do this.

— EMIL ZATOPEK

He had such unbelievable willpower that he could impose any burden of training he preferred upon himself.

— FRED WILT

I run and run, soft and squishy, easy rhythm, thinking of other things, and Dana comes home and there is yelling. Soapsuds down the hall! Soapsuds in my kitchen! But even she admit no one ever got shirts so white!

— EMIL ZATOPEK ON DOING LAUNDRY BY PUTTING IT IN THE BATHTUB
WITH SOAP AND WATER, PUTTING ON COMBAT BOOTS, AND RUNNING
ON IT

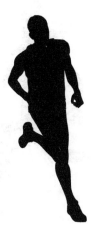

His enthusiasm, his friendliness, his love of life, shone through every movement. There is not and never was a greater man than Emil Zatopek.

— RON CLARKE

[B]ecoming rich was never my dream. For me it was best to have time for training, tracksuit for running, running shoes for training, stadium for training, all the nature and good food—that was enough.

— EMIL ZATOPEK

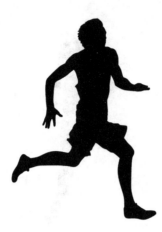

Before Zatopek, nobody realized it was humanly possible to train this hard.

— FRED WILT

Today, young boys and girls are not as active. By organizing competitions and training, you can grow in ability and health and disposition and have a healthy life. Or, we can live without productivity and training, and we'll go down.

— EMIL ZATOPEK

Everybody knows of his magnificent performances, but it would not be an overstatement to say that the personality of the man was even greater. In fact, to acknowledge that he was a unique figure in the history of distance running would be doing him an injustice. Much more simply, and more of the truth, Emil Zatopek himself is unique.

— RON CLARKE

CHAPTER NINE

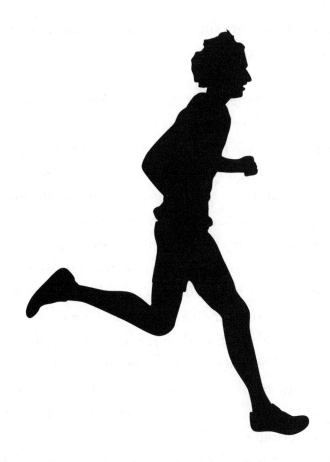

Life lessons in running

"I can't go on, I'll go on"

Although I can be highly competitive when properly self-motivated, sometimes I enter a road race for fun, happy to run with the back of the pack. Of course, all runs are supposed to be fun, but sometimes we lose sight of that fact in our constant desire to run faster, to prove something to ourselves and to others.

I have won four gold medals at the World Masters Championships and five silver and bronze, but sometimes I attend the bi-annual meet merely to signify my presence, not primed to succeed. At the Worlds in Rome one year, after competing on the track and in cross-country, I entered the marathon on the final day mainly as an excuse to run through the streets of the Eternal City, past monuments thousands of years old, without having to worry about being sideswiped by a Fiat. At one point toward the end of the race, I paused on an overlook that offered a view across the Tiber River toward St. Peter's Church. Then I continued to the finish line in the stadium used for the 1960 Olympic Games.

As I crossed the line, an Australian runner finishing in front of me turned and extended his hand, "That's the first time I ever beat you."

Taken by surprise by his comment, fatigued from the week's efforts, I responded with a remark ruder than needed: "You didn't beat me. You merely finished in front of me."

But the words ring true. We should not allow others to define our defeats and victories.

It does not matter how slowly you go so long as you do not stop.

— CONFUCIUS

You learn to speak by speaking, to study by studying, to run by running, to work by working; in just the same way, you learn to love by loving.

— ANATOLE FRANCE

Every time I fail I assume I will be a stronger person for it.

— JOAN BENOIT SAMUELSON

In our country, our sport is considered something of a miracle. When I won, many discovered that it was finally possible.

— JELENA PROKOPCUKA, 2005 AND 2006 WINNER OF THE NEW YORK CITY MARATHON, ON HER NATIVE LATVIA

In general, any form of exercise, if pursued continuously, will help train us in perseverance. Long-distance running is particularly good training in perseverance.

— MAO TSE-TUNG

Running is the greatest metaphor for life because you get out of it what you put into it.

— OPRAH WINFREY

Life is a marathon, not a sprint; pace yourself accordingly.

— AMBY BURFOOT, *THE RUNNER'S GUIDE TO THE MEANING OF LIFE*

I can't go on, I'll go on.

— SAMUEL BECKETT

Executives are like joggers. If you stop a jogger, he goes on running on the spot. If you drag an executive away from his business, he goes on running on the spot, pawing the ground, talking business. He never stops hurtling onwards, making decisions and executing them.

— JEAN BAUDRILLARD, *COOL MEMORIES*

Running actually helps with my studies. If I go out and run to the point of depletion and fatigue, all the gunk floating around in my head gets released, so I concentrate better when it's time to hit the books.

— RAY STEFFEN

Running has thrown me into adventures that I would otherwise have missed.

— BENJAMIN CHEEVER, *STRIDES*

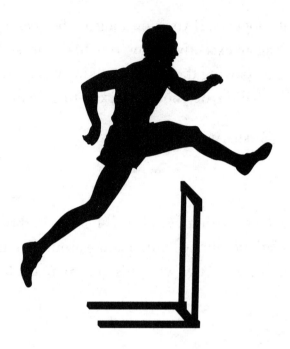

Sometimes runners think that they can do everything on their own, but support from others is essential, everyone from volunteers and spectators along the course to a helpful spouse who minds the kids while you train.

— HAL HIGDON

The other funny thing was the way he couldn't imagine himself ever walking again. It became automatic to run. Everything went by so much faster.

— RICHARD CHRISTIAN MATHESON, "THIRD WIND"

The race that I'm running now, I can never relax, never be finished. The day that I say I've got my addiction beat, I'll be in greater danger than when my leg got caught in [a farm accident when he was younger]. I can't let that day come.

— DICK BEARDSLEY

You can run full speed into a door that is closed or you can pull back just a little and go through the open door.

— JOHN BINGHAM, "THE DOORS," *RUNNERS WORLD*

Running taught me valuable lessons. In cross-country competition, training counted more than intrinsic ability, and I could compensate for a lack of natural aptitude with diligence and discipline. I applied this in everything I did.

— NELSON MANDELA

Running in the snow has its own special qualities—softness, quiet, the white landscape—and it can make you feel like a kid again.

— CLAIRE KOWALCHIK, *THE COMPLETE BOOK OF RUNNING FOR WOMEN*

As a boy, running was always pure joy for me. When I ran I would just let my mind wander and drift. But I would concentrate, too. I would imagine I could fly: *Run harder,* I would tell myself. *I know I can make a life of my own away from this farm.*

— HAILE GEBRSELASSIE, TWO-TIME OLYMPIC MEDALIST AND HOLDER OF THE WORLD RECORD FOR THE MARATHON (2:04:26)

The longer I run, the longer I practice (and I mean that in the meditative sense), the more mysterious the process becomes.

— ALISON TOWNSEND

Farming's a tough life. So is marathoning. Lots of hard work, little time off. Each life conditioned me for the other one.

— DICK BEARDSLEY

I view life as a series of training events building up to the big race and final finish line and I am always in training, always in the process of reaching the final goal.

— MATTHEW SHAFNER

Maybe people—both able-bodied and amputees—can look at me and say, "You know what? Life is tough, but if this guy can make it, then I can make it."

> — SCOTT RIGSBY, WHO IN 2007 BECAME THE FIRST DOUBLE-AMPUTEE TO COMPLETE AN IRONMAN TRIATHLON

Not only in running but in much of life is a sense of balance and proportion necessary.

> — CLARENCE DEMAR, 7-TIME WINNER OF THE BOSTON MARATHON

We may outrun
By violent swiftness that which we run at,
And lose by over-running.

> — SHAKESPEARE, *HENRY VIII*

Since I achieve something, running has exploded in my country.

— HAILE GEBRSELASSIE ON HIS NATIVE ETHIOPIA

———◆———

Run when I can, walk when I cannot run, and creep when I cannot walk.

— JOHN BUNYAN, *PILGRIM'S PROGRESS*

———◆———

[H]e, of all the people he'd ever known, was definitely climbing. Running had helped him get in the right frame of mind to do it. With each mileage barrier he broke, he was able to break greater barriers in life itself, especially his career.

— RICHARD CHRISTIAN MATHESON, "THIRD WIND"

———◆———

Each day [running] requires that I inhabit my body as completely as possible, surrender to change, and let that process work on me until I am not the tired and often dispirited woman who leave the house, but the one who returns enlivened, cheeks aflame, her mind swept clear as a Zen garden.

— ALISON TOWNSEND

Success rests in having the courage and endurance and, above all, the will to become the person you are, however peculiar that may be.

— GEORGE SHEEHAN

Running is the ultimate tortoise-and-hare activity because the tortoise wins all of the important races. Oh, sure, the hare might get a gold medal at the Olympics or Boston Marathon. But it's the tortoises who continue to run for decades and often even for a lifetime.

— AMBY BURFOOT, *THE PRINCIPLES OF RUNNING*

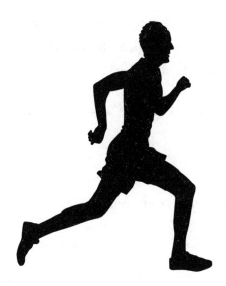

Runners are attuned to their bodies. They sense even tiny physical changes, the kinds that affect performance and general well-being. It was my running that first alerted me to my own illness [cancer], and my running that rehabilitated me from its ravages.

— FRED LEBOW

My wife says, "You always get your run in". . .Sometimes I wish I devoted more time to my family like a lot of others who are my age, but running has changed my life so much.

— *BILL RODGERS' LIFETIME RUNNING PLAN*

Pain is inevitable. Suffering is optional.

— ANONYMOUS

If a man coaches himself, then he has only himself to blame when he is beaten.

— ROGER BANNISTER

He ran another hundred yards and he prayed, "Please let me just finish. I don't want to beat anybody. All I want to do is just finish." Because somewhere inside him was the idea that if he could endure it just this one time, then maybe he would get his fair chance, when he could really do something, tomorrow.

— JAMES BUECHLER, "JOHN SOBIESKI BURNS"

It's not about speed and gold medals. It's about refusing to be stopped.

— AMBY BURFOOT

In every little village in the world there are great potential champions who only need motivation, development, and good exercise evaluation.

— ARTHUR LYDIARD

Running is a lot like life. Only 10 percent of it is exciting. 90 percent of it is slog and drudge.

> — DAVE BEDFORD, ENGLISH DISTANCE RUNNER WHO OCCASIONALLY PUT IN 200 MILES A WEEK IN TRAINING

Ask yourself: "Can I give more?" The answer is usually yes.

> — PAUL TERGAT

Pain is temporary, but pride lasts forever.

> — ANONYMOUS

Fear is the strongest driving-force in competition. Not fear of one's opponent, but of the skill and high standard which he represents; fear, too, of not acquitting oneself well.

> — FRANZ STAMPFL

[A]round a tight bend, take off like holy hell.

— JOHN TREACY

⬥

You can't stop the exterior aging. . . . It's because of health and fitness, and what I eat, and exercise especially, that inside I feel really young.

— PRISCILLA WELCH

⬥

Ignore, then, whether you are tall and thin or short and stocky—whether they laughed at you at home (where they are often unkind) or at school (where they *are* mostly blind, anyway). Indeed—to hell with the lot of them if you "feel" you can do it.

— PERCY CERUTTY

⬥

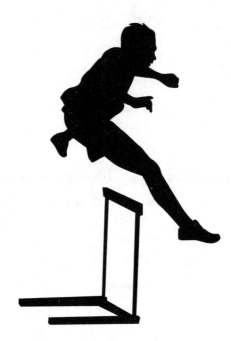

It's at the borders of pain and suffering that the men are separated from the boys.

— EMIL ZATOPEK

Every day you have to test yourself. If you don't, it's a wasted day.

— TERRY BUTTS, MARINE CORPS MALE ATHLETE OF THE YEAR

Success rests in having the courage and endurance and, above all, the will to become the person you are, however peculiar that may be.

— GEORGE SHEEHAN

We must all suffer one of two things: the pain of discipline or the pain of regret or disappointment.

— JIM ROHN

Running along a beach at sunrise with no other footprints in the sand, you realize the vastness of creation, your own insignificant space in the plan [. . .] your own creatureliness and how much you owe to the supreme body, the God that brought all this beauty and harmony into being.

— SISTER MARION IRVINE

[T]he discipline it took to train has entered all facets of my life. I am more focused, get more done during the day.

— MATTHEW SHAFNER

As runners, we all go through many transitions—transitions that closely mimic the larger changes we experience in a lifetime. First, we try to run faster. Then we try to run harder. Then we learn to accept ourselves and our limitations, and at last, we can appreciate the true joy and meaning of running.

— AMBY BURFOOT

I had to do something to shake up my life and get back some sense of control and trust in the world and along the way fill the hollow space. I needed to rebel against those negative forces, to scream so loud and for so long that the anger living inside me would evacuate forever. But instead of screaming, I ran.

— GAIL W. KISLEVITZ ON RUNNING AFTER HER DIAGNOSIS WITH SKIN CANCER

We went through stages on what to do. My first response was, "Nothing is worth the loss of human life." Then I thought that by stopping the games we'd be doing exactly what the terrorists wanted.

— FRANK SHORTER ON THE 1972 MUNICH OLYMPICS, AT WHICH PALESTINIAN TERRORISTS TOOK HOSTAGES

I don't believe in striving for extremely fast times and intense levels of competition. I have witnessed the demise of an entire generation of hotshots.

— JOHN BABINGTON, LIBERTY ATHLETIC CLUB COACH AND ASSISTANT COACH FOR THE 1996 OLYMPIC WOMEN'S TRACK-AND-FIELD TEAM

Once the stopwatch was important for checking splits or a training pace; now I check my watch to pick up the children at school or to meet the babysitter.

— JOAN BENOIT SAMUELSON

I have learned that there is no failure in running, or in life, as long as you keep moving.

— AMBY BURFOOT

Speed is often confused with insight. When I start running earlier than the others, I appear faster.

— JOHAN CRUIJFF

One chance is all you need.

— JESSE OWENS

Believe in your program, do what you can, be prepared for life's surprises, expect the unexpected.

— LORRAINE MOLLER ON TRAINING

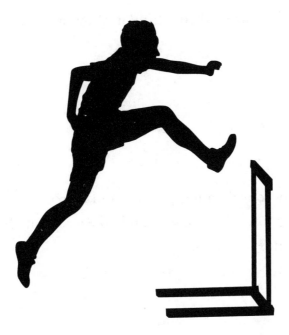

There are those of us who are always about to live. We are waiting until things change, until there is more time, until we are less tired, until we get a promotion, until we settle down . . . until, until, until. It always seems as if there is some major event that must occur in our lives before we begin living.

— GEORGE SHEEHAN

Find the good. It's all around you. Find it, showcase it, and you'll start believing in it.

— Jesse Owens

I advise you to say your dream is possible and then overcome all inconveniences, ignore all the hassles and take a running leap through the hoop, even if it is in flames.

— Les Brown

Champions are made when no one is watching.

— Anonymous

The long run puts the tiger in the cat.

— Bill Squires

It's like people always say, "Well, does sport teach you anything in life?" It teaches you certain things, but it doesn't teach you about other things. It doesn't teach, as I say, very much about marriage, very much about how to make a living, any of those things.

— GEORGE PLIMPTON

A runner must run with dreams in his heart, not money in his pocket.

— EMIL ZATOPEK

Know yourself, so you may live that life peculiar to you, the one and only life you were born to live. Know yourself, that you may perfect your body and find your play.

— GEORGE SHEEHAN

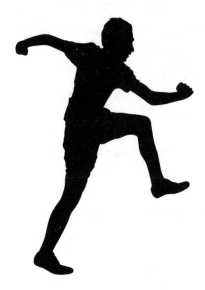

You only ever grow as a human being if you're outside your comfort zone.

— PERCY CERUTTY

I cannot have survival as my only goal. That would be too boring. My goal is to come back in my best running form. It is good for me to have that goal; it will help me.

— LUDMILLA ENGQUIST, RUSSIAN-SWEDISH OLYMPIAN WHO WAS DIAGNOSED WITH BREAST CANCER IN 1999

When I came back, after all those stories about Hitler and his snub, I came back to my native country, and I could not ride in the front of the bus. I had to go to the back door. I couldn't live where I wanted. Now what's the difference.

— Jesse Owens

I think that carrying a baby inside you is like running as fast as you can. It feels like finally letting go and filling yourself up to the widest limits.

— Quoted in *Ourselves and Our Children*

The sportsman, the real sportsman, knows what is inside him.

— Emil Zatopek

What fun is it? Why all that hard, exhausting work? Where does it get you? Where's the good of it? It is one of the strange ironies of this strange life that those who work the hardest, who subject themselves to the strictest discipline, who give up certain pleasurable things in order to achieve a goal, are the happiest.

— BRUTUS HAMILTON, COACH OF THE 1948 U.S. OLYMPIC TRACK AND FIELD TEAM

———

It is distance, not speed, that holds the answers. The reward comes with crossing and confronting the boundaries of fatigue.

— JOHN BINGHAM, *THE COURAGE TO START*

———

Our greatest glory is not never falling, but in rising every time we fall.

— CONFUCIUS

———

Stadiums are for spectators. We runners have Nature, and that is much better.

— JUHA VAATAINEN

Ξ

You're just running. You're not putting together business plans, solving quadratic equations, or trying to keep your drive from slicing off the fairway.

— AMBY BURFOOT, *THE RUNNER'S GUIDE TO THE MEANING OF LIFE*

Ξ

We never try to put ceilings on anyone. Years ago certain records were unattainable, but it happens. In any given situation in any given time, anything can happen.

— SUE HUMPHREY

Ξ

No matter who we are, at some point we are all first-time marathoners. . .We all set goals for ourselves. We all work hard. We all seek to be surrounded by others who will encourage and support us.

— GRETE WAITZ AND GLORIA AVERBUCH, *RUN YOUR FIRST MARATHON*

Now if you are going to win any battle you have to do one thing. You have to make the mind run the body. Never let the body tell the mind what to do. The body will always give up. It is always tired morning, noon, and night. But the body is never tired if the mind is not tired. When you were younger the mind could make you dance all night, and the body was never tired. You've always got to make the mind take over and keep going.

— GEORGE S. PATTON, U.S. ARMY GENERAL AND 1912 OLYMPIAN

Let him that would move the world first move himself.

— SOCRATES

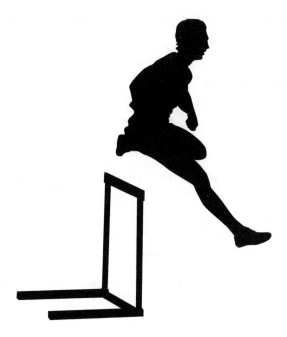

Taking charge of your body can help you take charge of your life. And that power can help you go wherever you want to go, every single day.

> — CHERYL BRIDGES TREWORGY, MEMBER OF FIVE U.S. WORLD CROSS-COUNTRY TEAMS

One of the great benefits of running is that it teaches us to value the individual—*our self*.

> — AMBY BURFOOT, *THE RUNNER'S GUIDE TO THE MEANING OF LIFE*

The most important thing I learned [from running] is that there is only one runner in this race, and that is me.

— GEORGE SHEEHAN

Have a dream, make a plan, go for it. You'll get there, I promise.

— ZOE KOPLOWITZ

All records fall.

— AMBY BURFOOT, *THE RUNNER'S GUIDE TO THE MEANING OF LIFE*

It is not necessary for me that you are running. But if you don't run, I'm sure you'll be sorry for it later on.

— HUSBAND OF FANNY BLANKERS-KOEN, RESPONDING TO HER REQUEST THAT THEY LEAVE THE 1948 OLYMPICS TO SEE THEIR CHILDREN. SHE WON FOUR GOLD MEDALS AT THOSE GAMES.

Leading is the best way to stay out of trouble.

— MARY DECKER SLANEY

A run is most meaningful and enjoyable when it exists for its own sake, when it doesn't feel the pressure of a ticking stopwatch. The same goes for most other activities.

— AMBY BURFOOT, *THE RUNNER'S GUIDE TO THE MEANING OF LIFE*

I like to make people stop and say, "I've never seen anyone run like that before!" It's more than just a race, it's a style. It's doing something better than anyone else.

— STEVE PREFONTAINE

CHAPTER TEN

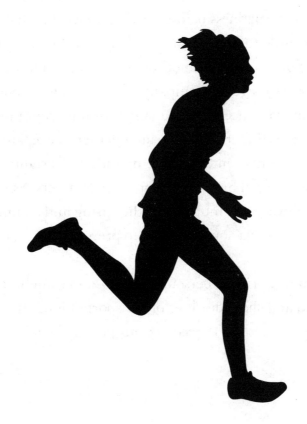

Motivation and inspiration

"Just Run"

As runners we often run alone, climbing out of bed early, donning our shoes and rushing out the door into the darkness of a winter morning to claim our moment of madness before heading to work, what we do when not running. Too little time to call a friend and meet on a corner to break the solitariness of our pursuit. Out of my way, World: Here I come!

Yet other times we crave the company of others. This is one of the main appeals, I am convinced, of the many training programs so popular in large cities, where runners meet to run together to prepare themselves for some major running event, usually a marathon. Certainly this is true with the class offered by the Chicago Area Runners Association, where on a typical weekend morning in the spring and summer several thousand will gather in various locations to prepare for that city's fall marathon.

Thus, sometimes we run as personal entities, and sometimes we gather in groups to bond and share our love of the sport of long distance runner. We can be alone or together. It becomes our personal choice.

You train best where you are the happiest.

— FRANK SHORTER

⸺◆⸺

This is what really matters: running. This is where I know where I am.

— STEVE JONES

⸺◆⸺

Tell the truth and run.

— YUGOSLAVIAN PROVERB

⸺◆⸺

[Y]ou need to start slowly, yes, but you do need to make an effort, you do need to push at times, a little beyond the point of comfort.

— *RUNNING FOR DUMMIES*

⸺◆⸺

For the elite, fear of losing a race is often the most powerful motivator.

— AMBY BURFOOT

———◆———

Matter is arbitrary. It is your will against mine, your spirit against mine. Everything depends on the will.

— BRIAN GANVILLE, "THE OLYMPIAN"

———◆———

The law of nature is, do the thing, and you shall have the power: but they who do not the thing have not the power.

— RALPH WALDO EMERSON

———◆———

God determines how fast you're going to run; I can help only with the mechanics.

— BILL BOWERMAN

———◆———

Coaches are okay, I guess, but I prefer to do things my own way.

— JACK FOSTER

Among the strong, there are the strongest, and behind the able, there are even abler.

— CHINESE PROVERB

The thinking must be done first, before training begins.

— PETER COE

Run when you can, walk if you have to, crawl if you must; just never give up.

— DEAN KARNAZES

Every athlete has doubts. Elite runners in particular are insecure people. You need someone to affirm that what you are doing is right.

— LYNN JENNINGS

Act like a horse. Be dumb. Just run.

— JUMBO ELLIOTT

[Famous runners'] stories ignite and shape our young strainings.

— KENNY MOORE

When I crossed the finish line in first place at the World Masters Championships in Finland, I knelt and kissed the track. It embarrassed my wife sitting in the stands, but it was the track that had carried me to victory.

— HAL HIGDON

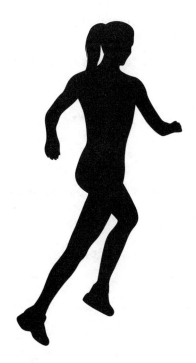

The Empire is saved. Roar, Lion, Roar! There's been nothing to compare to this since the destruction of the Spanish Armada. Let the Aga Khan take such satisfaction as he may from his Epsom Derby winners. Let Ben Hogan have the British Open title and welcome. England has the four-minute mile.

— RED SMITH, "EMPIRE REBORN," *INTERNATIONAL HERALD TRIBUNE*, MAY 8, 1954

It is not the doing of it that really counts, but doing it FIRST.

— NORRIS MCWHIRTER IN *ATHLETICS WORLD*, MAY 1954

Whether you jog or run is a question of semantics more than commitment or ability.

— MARC BLOOM, *THE RUNNER'S BIBLE*

Fate is never too generous—even to its favorites. Rarely do the gods grant a mortal more than one immortal deed.

— STEFAN ZWEIG

You're ready for new challenges, for whatever life brings, and you run like a deer across the tops of the hills.

— *THE RUNNER'S BOOK OF DAILY INSPIRATION*, KEVIN NELSON

———◆———

Winning my first World Cross Country title made me feel invincible. Winning my second one made me feel even more that way. If I win a third, I feel like I can run through a brick wall.

— LYNN JENNINGS

———◆———

A great coach is an artist. You have to be creative, and you have to capture enough kids to create your artwork.

— PAT TYSON

———◆———

Believe that you can run farther or faster. Believe that you're young enough, old enough, strong enough, and so on to accomplish everything you want to do. Don't let worn out beliefs stop you from moving beyond yourself.

— JOHN BINGHAM, "TOOLS AND RULES," *RUNNERS WORLD*

One man's (or woman's) motivation is another's black hole.

— AMBY BURFOOT

To keep your motivation high, use mental stimuli. Find out what gets you psyched, and surround yourself with it; posters, sayings, photos, running magazines, videos.

— GRETE WAITZ

Generally slow running is considered jogging, but I think you're better off considering yourself a runner from the start.

— MARC BLOOM, *THE RUNNER'S BIBLE*

If you need help getting motivated, turn to fellow runners. Often, they have been there, done that and can help move you along.

— HAL HIGDON

Everybody and their mother knows you don't train hard on Friday, the day before a race. But a lot of runners will over-train on Thursday if left on their own. Thursday is the most dangerous day of the week.

— MARTY STERN, VILLANOVA WOMEN'S TRACK AND CROSS-COUNTRY COACH

Some people say, "Oh, you're doing only 10-minute miles; you're just a jogger," but it feels like running to me. If you say to yourself you're a runner, you feel more confident, more powerful.

— KATHY DOUKAS

Fear of trying causes paralysis. Trying causes only trembling and sweating.

— MASON COOLEY

Running doesn't have to be monotonous if you put a little imagination into your step.

— CLAIRE KOWALCHIK, *THE COMPLETE BOOK OF RUNNING FOR WOMEN*

In order to cash in on all the training, get the rest. If you can't run as fast as you want to, you haven't rested enough.

— TED CORBITT

Remember, the feeling you get from a good run is far better than the feeling you get from sitting around wishing you were running.

— SARAH CONDOR

You can't flirt with the track. You must marry it.

— BILL EASTON

There are few instincts more natural than the body in full motion as it races across a field or through the trees.

— NEAL BASCOMB, *THE PERFECT MILE*

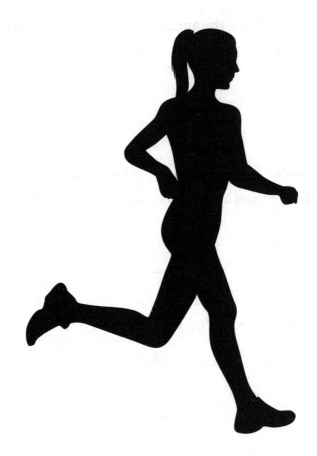

Learn to run when feeling the pain: then push harder.

— WILLIAM SIGEI

"We can lay it on the line, bust a gut, show them a clean pair of heels. We can sprint the turn on a spring breeze and feel the winter leave our feet! We can, by God, let our demons loose and just wail on!"

— QUENTIN CASSIDY IN *ONCE A RUNNER* BY JOHN L. PARKER, JR.

Your training partner's name is pain. You start out trying to ignore him. Can't do it. You attempt to reason with him. No way. You try to strike a bargain. Ha. You plead. You say "Please stop, please go away. I promise never ever to do this again if you just leave me alone." But he won't. Pain only climbs off if you do. Then you're beaten.

— SCOTT MARTIN

When the desire strikes, simply put on a pair of shorts and a T-shirt, lace up your running shoes, and head down the road, up a trail, or through an open field.

— CLAIRE KOWALCHIK, *THE COMPLETE BOOK OF RUNNING FOR WOMEN*

Men's actions are too strong for them. Show me a man who has acted, and who has not been the victim and slave of his action.

— RALPH WALDO EMERSON

Some days it's not dangerous and some days it is. But I'm staying here to recover and I want to start training again.

— LUKE KIBET, MARATHON GOLD-MEDALIST AT THE 2007
WORLD CHAMPIONSHIPS IN ATHLETICS, SPEAKING AFTER BEING
ATTACKED DURING THE VIOLENCE THAT ENGULFED HIS NATIVE
KENYA FOLLOWING THE DISPUTED ELECTIONS AT THE END
OF 2007

[M]otivation is a skill. It can be learned and practiced.

— AMBY BURFOOT

There comes a time late in the afternoon when the light is just so and my circadian rhythms are at exactly a certain point, when the only solid thought in my mind is to *run*.

— ALISON TOWNSEND

In the 30 years I've been a runner I've run more than 150,000 miles. Still, some of the hardest steps I take are those first few getting out the door for daily runs.

— *BILL RODGERS' LIFETIME RUNNING PLAN*

You can't talk yourself into shape. Either you can do it or you can't.

— FRANK SHORTER

Knowing that I've got a marathon down the road is what gets me to lace up my shoes and head out the door each morning.

— JULIE DWORSCHACK

My coworkers and non-running friends, even my husband, tend to think I am weird for running. I get tired of defending myself, of trying to make them understand what it means to me. With my running friends, I don't have to go through all that.

— KIM AHRENS

I trotted on along the edge of a field bordered by the sunken lane, smelling green grass and honeysuckle, and I felt as though I came from a long line of whippets trained to run on two legs.

— ALAN SILLITOE, "THE LONELINESS OF THE LONG-DISTANCE RUNNER"

I don't believe in burnout. I believe in losing your appetite.

— PAT TYSON

Your shoes are only as good as the laces they're attached to.

— GREG SAMPSON

Some people endure pain better than others. All things considered, the ability to withstand—or even deny—pain would seem to be a valuable ally for the long distance runner in search of significant improvement. In truth, it is probably a double-edged sword, since medical experts tell us that pain is the body's warning signal to back off, and that to ignore such schedules is to roll the dice with both body and mind.

— MARK WILL-WEBER

Top results are reached only through pain. But eventually you like this pain. You'll find the more difficulties you have on the way, the more you will enjoy your success.

— Juha "The Cruel" Väätäinen

Nothing's better than the wind to your back, the sun in front of you, and your friends beside you.

— Aaron Douglas Trimble

Those who say that I will lose and am finished will have to run over my body to beat me.

— Said Aouita

Beyond the sky there is more sky; beyond one person there are others as well.

— CHINESE PROVERB

I believe you'll develop speed via strength work, which includes hill running, or running hilly courses, as the Kenyans do on a steady basis.

— BILL RODGERS

A runner's creed: I will win; if I cannot win, I shall be second; if I cannot be second, I shall be third; if I cannot place at all, I shall still do my best.

— KEN DOHERTY

Any idiot can train himself into the ground; the trick is working in training to get gradually stronger.

— KEITH BRANTLY

"Winning" is an elusive if not irrelevant goal to most runners.

— *RUNNING FOR DUMMIES*

The introduction of resistance in form of sand and hill is too important to be ignored.

— PERCY CERUTTY

The Truth is that Running Hurts. No one gets faster without meeting their personal pain barrier straight on.

— "MANCIATA," WWW.10KTRUTH.COM

I listened to the rhythm of my breath, which was unsteady as early as twelve miles into the race. By fifteen miles, lots of women were passing me and I understood that I might not make it. Without despair I continued step by step.

— MAX APPLE, "CARBO-LOADING"

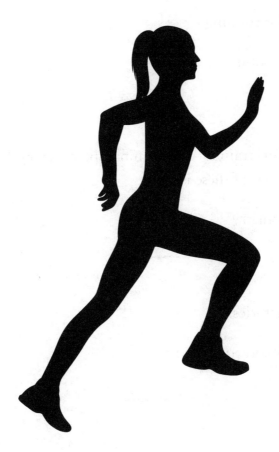

If you set your aim too high and don't fulfill it, then your enthusiasm turns to bitterness. Try for a goal that's reasonable, and then gradually raise it.

— EMIL ZATOPEK

Hills are terrific for running.

— BILL RODGERS

———◆———

The five S's of sports training are: stamina, speed, strength, skill, and spirit; but the greatest of these is spirit.

— KEN DOHERTY

———◆———

Recognize your victories.

— JOAN BENOIT SAMUELSON

———◆———

Running well is a matter of having the patience to persevere when we are tired and not expecting instant results.

— ROBERT DE CASTELLA

———◆———

Heart has nothing to do with it. In the final straight, *everyone* has heart.

— JOHN L. PARKER, JR.,*ONCE A RUNNER*

———◆———

Make the expectations lively enough, and action will follow.

— MASON COOLEY

———◆———

There is a great advantage in training under unfavorable conditions. It is better to train under bad conditions, for the difference is then a tremendous relief in a race.

— EMIL ZATOPEK

———◆———

Nobody is going to win a 5,000-meter race after running an easy two miles.

— STEVE PREFONTAINE

———◆———

Running with others can help get you out when you might otherwise blow it off.

— Frank Shorter

⎯⎯◈⎯⎯

Avoid running at all times.

— Satchel Paige

⎯⎯◈⎯⎯

[R]unning is a year-round sport and you train for all conditions, so you sort of have to be mentally prepared, physically sort of used to it.

— Bill Rodgers

⎯⎯◈⎯⎯

But if you can find that spot—I suppose it's like running—I used to be a swimmer and swim laps, and you just have to be there with what you're doing.

— Bruce Nauman

⎯⎯◈⎯⎯

Encourage kids to enjoy running and play in athletics. Don't force them to run too much competition.

— Arthur Lydiard

———◆———

In the seventies, I was a school teacher and trained at 5 AM and 5 PM. During wintertime, I never saw the sun.

— Tom Fleming (one of the all time great American runners. Won the New York City Marathon twice, took second at Boston two times)

———◆———

The world leaves no track in space, and the greatest action of man no mark in the vast idea.

— Ralph Waldo Emerson

———◆———

Over the first stile, without trying, I was still nearly in the lead but one; and if any of you want tips about running, never be in a hurry, and never let any of the other runners know you are in a hurry even if you are.

— ALAN SILLITOE, *THE LONELINESS OF THE LONG-DISTANCE RUNNER*

Commitment to the body machine. It was as critical as the commitment to the goal itself.

— RICHARD CHRISTIAN MATHESON, "THIRD WIND"

Pretend you are a gazelle," he says, "a gazelle along the verdant banks of the ancient Tiber, or a sleek antelope galloping toward some lush African watering place."

— MAX APPLE, "CARBO-LOADING"

Looking forward to something is much more fun than looking back at something—and much more constructive.

— HORTENSE ODLUM

⬥

The young man who meant to be a fast runner and tireless walker was enjoined to go through a course of physic taking, between an ounce and a half and two ounces of Glauber salts *[laxatives]* every four days until three doses had been administered.

— WALTER THOM, *PEDESTRIANISM* (1813)

⬥

May is a very early time in the year and the weather is usually bad. You cannot run a fast mile race if there is a strong wind, because it makes your running uneven.

— ROGER BANNISTER

⬥

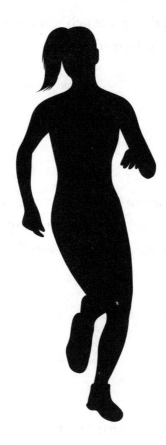

Running in your dreams may also symbolize the energy levels, the strength, or the force that you have to get through life.

— SILVANA AMAR, *THE BEDSIDE DREAM DICTIONARY*

I have my routine. I'm running three or four miles a day.

— DIRK BENEDICT

To keep motivated, I started swearing at my husband for getting me into this mess in the first place.

— GRETE WAITZ ON HER FIRST TIME RUNNING THE NEW YORK CITY MARATHON, IN 1978

I believe 100 percent in continued running after forty, and racing too, if one so desires.

— BILL RODGERS

How can one learn to know oneself? Never by introspection, rather by action.

— JOHANN WOLFGANG VON GOETHE

When I was young, I was too slow. I thought I must learn to run fast by practicing to run fast, so I ran 100 meters fast 20 times. Then I came back slow, slow, slow. People said, "Emil, you are crazy. You are training like a sprinter."

— EMIL ZATOPEK

Somewhere in the world someone is training when you are not. When you race him, he will win.

— TOM FLEMING'S BOSTON MARATHON TRAINING MOTTO

Runners like to train 100 miles per week because it's a round number. But I think 88 is a lot rounder.

— DON KARDONG

[An athlete should walk] from twenty to twenty-four miles a day. He must rise at five in the morning, run half a mile at the top of his speed up-hill, and then walk six miles at a moderate pace, coming in about seven to breakfast, which should consist of beefsteaks or mutton-chops underdone, with stale bread and old beer. After breakfast, he must again walk six miles at a moderate pace, and at twelve lie down without his clothes for half an hour.

— WALTER THOM

A change of pace in terms of your running pace will give you strength psychologically.

— BILL RODGERS

Some people can't figure out what I'm doing. It's not a walk-hop, it's not a trot, it's running, or as close as I can get to running, and it's harder than doing it on two legs. It makes me mad when people call this a walk. If I was walking it wouldn't be anything.

— TERRY FOX

There's no such thing as bad weather, just soft people.

— BILL BOWERMAN

If one can stick to the training throughout the many long years, then will power is no longer a problem. It's raining? That doesn't matter. I am tired? That's besides the point. It's simply that I just have to.

— EMIL ZATOPEK

Sometimes . . . an injury may be due to increased running, fatigue, sickness, etc. and have nothing at all to do with your shoe.

— BILL RODGERS

He that would be a great man must learn to turn every accident to some advantage.

— FRANCOIS DUC DE LA ROCHEFOUCAULD

Experience has taught me how important it is to just keep going, focusing on running fast and relaxed. Eventually [pain] passes and the flow returns. It's part of racing.

— FRANK SHORTER

When a person trains once, nothing happens. When a person forces himself to do a thing a hundred or a thousand times, then he certainly has developed in more ways than physical.

— EMIL ZATOPEK

During the hard training phase, never be afraid to take a day off. If your legs are feeling unduly stiff and sore, rest; if you are at all sluggish, rest; in fact, if in doubt, rest.

— BRUCE FORDYCE

If you train hard, you'll not only be hard, you'll be hard to beat.

— HERSCHEL WALKER

Train, don't strain.

— ARTHUR LYDIARD

There are twenty ways of going to a point, and one is the shortest; but set out at once on one.

— RALPH WALDO EMERSON

I tell the kids to have "wide eyes," to run light as a feather, to get high on their toes, and to dig deep, dig deep, dig deep!

— PAT TYSON

Let your running lead you to your diet.

— BILL RODGERS

No amount of junk miles, fun runs or affirmations are going to get you over the hill at the five-mile mark in a 10k. However, what will pull you through is solid prep with hard hill runs and interval work.

— MANCIATA

Dwell on the positive, but have controlled, passionate anger.

— PAT TYSON

Run hard, be strong, think big!

— PERCY CERUTTY

I believe in keeping running simple and, in regard to shoes, that would mean no gimmicks, unnecessary cushioning, etc.

— BILL RODGERS

Don't attack a hill from the very bottom—it's bigger than you are!

— HARRY GROVES, PENN STATE COACH

See what you are about to do as a thing that has already been accomplished; it will in fact help you do it. The race will already be run before you run it.

— *THE RUNNER'S BOOK OF DAILY INSPIRATION*, KEVIN NELSON

You would fain be victor at the Olympic games, you say. Yes, but weigh the conditions, weigh the consequences; then and then only, lay to your hand if it be for your profit.

— EPICTETUS

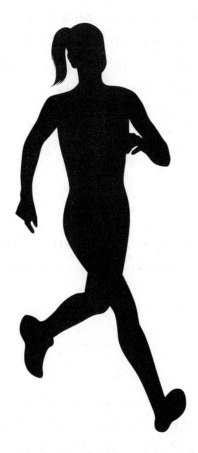

He was giving all he had, in the only way he knew; he was going to run as fast as he could for as long as he could, and let it go at that.

— EDDY ORCUTT, "WHEELBARROW"

Physiologists and high-performance trainers understand now that the concept of 110 percent is no longer a smart way to train. Give 110 percent, and you won't build your body up, but actually break it down. And be no good to yourself or anyone else.

— SALLY JENKINS, THE *WASHINGTON POST*

Thus I urge you to go on to your greatness if you believe it is in you. Think deeply and separate what you wish from what you are prepared to do.

— PERCY CERUTTY

The more I talk to athletes, the more convinced I become that the method of training is relatively unimportant. There are many ways to the top, and the training method you choose is just the one that suits you best. No, the important thing is the attitude of the athlete, the desire to get to the top.

— HERB ELLIOTT

My lover has the most beautiful body in the world. Because she runs. I fell in love with her because she had the most beautiful body I had ever seen.

> — SARA MAITLAND, "THE LOVELINESS OF THE LONG-DISTANCE RUNNER"

Training is principally an act of faith. The athlete must believe in its efficacy; he must believe that through training he will become fitter and stronger; that by constant repetition of the same movements he will become more skillfull and his muscles more relaxed.

> — FRANZ STAMPFL, *On Running*

You must live by rule, submit to diet, abstain from dainty meats, exercise your body perforce at stated hours, in heat or in cold; drink no cold water, nor, it may be, wine. In a word, you must surrender yourself wholly to your trainer, as though to a physician.

> — EPICECTUS

Most track coaches kind of criticize my short gait, and it's so funny, because as a little five-year-old, when I won my first race, I had this huge, gaping gait and I wore these boots.

— GABE JENNINGS

Running in the correct shoe is key.

— BILL RODGERS

Talk to your body, and if you're ready to make a commitment, have a go at it.

— PRISCILLA WELCH

They say you can't run away from your troubles. I say that you can.

— JOHN BINGHAM, *THE COURAGE TO START*

Even during the height of the war in neighboring Bosnia, Dejan Nikolic persisted in putting on the Belgrade Marathon. . . . [D]espite the difficulties, Nikolic insisted that the marathon must continue because, he said, he wanted "to show the world that runners have so much in common."

— Michael Sandrock

If the coach cannot do it, he cannot "teach" it—only talk about it.

— Percy Cerutty

The Zulu warrior women could run fifty miles a day and fight at the end of it. Fifty miles together, perfectly in step, so the veldt drummed with it. Did their hearts beat as one? My heart can beat with theirs, slow and strong and efficient—pumping energy.

— Sara Maitland, "The Loveliness of the Long-Distance Runner"

When her last child is off to school, we don't want the talented woman wasting her time in work far below her capacity. We want her to come out running.

— MARY INGRAHAM BUNTING, THEN PRESIDENT OF RADCLIFFE COLLEGE (1961)

There. I've done my best. If that won't do, I shall have to wait until I can do better.

— VICTOR HEERMAN

My dad had me do these drills while I was running to school, and just on the field, he's like, "Sprinters need to have quick steps. You need to get as much turnover as possible,' and he had me do these drills, like, 'Dah-dah dah-dah dah-dah dah-dah" as quick as I could go, and I, like, really consciously shortened my gait. I still remember this as a little kid, thinking, "OK, to be a sprinter, I need to have a short gait."

— GABE JENNINGS

Even a toad has four ounces of strength.

— CHINESE PROVERB

—◦—

Sometimes you're overwhelmed when a thing comes, and you do not realize the magnitude of the affair at that moment. When you get away from it, you wonder, did it really happen to you.

— MARIAN ANDERSON

—◦—

Honors to me now are not what they once were.

— CHESTER A. ARTHUR

—◦—

There are two great rules in life, the one general and the other particular. The first is that everyone can in the end get what he wants if he only tries. This is the general rule. The particular rule is that every individual is more or less of an exception to the general rule.

— SAMUEL BUTLER

—◦—

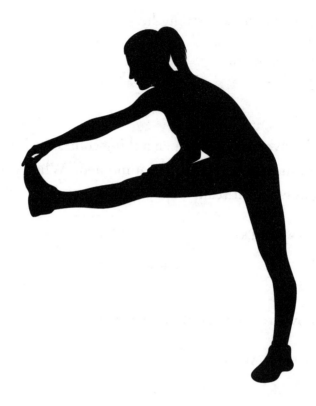

Attaining even mediocrity is often a struggle.

— MASON COOLEY

The end crowneth the work.

— ELIZABETH I

❖

Soon there will be nothing truly profound that is not achieved by everyone, and of the difficult things in this world only one will be left: simplicity.

— FRANZ GRILLPARZER

❖

I'm not out there sweating for three hours every day just to find out what it feels like to sweat.

— MICHAEL JORDAN

❖

Man can acquire accomplishments or he can become an animal, whichever he wants. God makes the animals, man makes himself.

— GEORG CHRISTOPH LICHTENBERG

❖

Man is always more than he can know of himself; consequently, his accomplishments, time and again, will come as a surprise to him.

— GOLO MANN

He who attains his ideal, thereby also transcends it.

— FRIEDRICH NIETZSCHE

One of the greatest satisfactions one can ever have, comes from the knowledge that he can do some one thing superlatively well.

— HORTENSE ODLUM

When you've trained as best you can and you know your competition has done the same, nothing really matters but your mental strength and your belief.

— FLORENCE GRIFFITH JOYNER

I'm overwhelmed by the strength of my body and the power of my mind. For one moment, just one second, I feel immortal.

— DIANA NYAD

If one has determination, then things will get done.

— CHINESE PROVERB

So many worlds, so much to do,
So little done, such things to be.

— ALFRED TENNYSON

I am more fond of achieving than striving.

— CAROLYN WELLS

When it looks at great accomplishments, the world, bent on simplifying its images, likes best to look at the dramatic, picturesque moments experienced by its heroes. . . . But the no less creative years of preparation remain in the shadow.

— STEFAN ZWEIG

Action is only coarsened thought—thought becomes concrete, obscure, and unconscious.

— HENRI-FRÉDÉRIC AMIEL

Action without a name, a "who" attached to it, is meaningless.

— HANNAH ARENDT

He who desires but acts not, breeds pestilence.

— WILLIAM BLAKE

It is vain to say human beings ought to be satisfied with tranquility: they must have action; and they will make it if they cannot find it

— CHARLOTTE BRONTE

Fruitless striving breeds less despair than inaction.

— MASON COOLEY

Good thoughts are no better than good dreams, unless they be executed.

— RALPH WALDO EMERSON

Action is character.

— F. SCOTT FITZGERALD

The safest thing is always to try to convert everything that is in us and around us into action.

— JOHANN WOLFGANG VON GOETHE

In our era, the road to holiness necessarily passes through the world of action.

— DAG HAMMARSKJOLD

Two possibilities: making oneself infinitely small or being so. The second is perfection, that is to say, inactivity, the first is beginning, that is to say, action.

— FRANZ KAFKA

Keep always busy so that the devil will find you always engaged.

— JEROME

In the end, I think you really only get as far as you're allowed to get.

— GAYLE GARDNER

Possess the spirit of independence.

— MARIA STEWART

No advantages in this world are pure and unmixed.

— DAVID HUME

An adventure is only an inconvenience rightly considered. An inconvenience is only an adventure wrongly considered.

— GILBERT KEITH CHESTERTON

"Why not?" is a slogan for an interesting life.

— MASON COOLEY

The search for adventure is the vent which Destiny offers.

— RALPH WALDO EMERSON

My love of running is a feeling every woman can experience.

— JOAN BENOIT SAMUELSON

We are the men of intrinsic value, who can strike our fortunes out of ourselves.

— GEORGE FARQUHAR

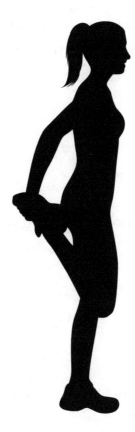

Two deep human desires were at war . . . the longing for stability, for form, for permanence, which in its essence is the desire for death, and the opposing hunger for movement, change, instability, and risk, which are life.

— ROSE WILDER LANE

There are two kinds of adventurers: Those who go truly hoping to find adventure and those who go secretly hoping they won't.

— WILLIAM TROGDON

Living each day as a preparation for the next is an exciting way to live.

— HORTENSE ODLUM

If we do not find anything very pleasant, at least we shall find something new.

— VOLTAIRE

If we didn't live venturously, plucking the wild goat by the beard, and trembling over precipices, we should never be depressed, I've no doubt; but already should be faded, fatalistic and aged.

— VIRGINIA WOOLF

Not being able to control events, I control myself; and I adapt myself to them, if they do not adapt themselves to me.

— MICHEL DE MONTAIGNE

Impossible? . . . Napoleon said that word is not French.

— P. J. WOLFSON

I certainly admire people who do things.

— RAYMOND CHANDLER

Maturity involves being honest and true to oneself, making decisions based on a conscious internal process, assuming responsibility for one's decisions, having healthy relationships with others and developing one's own true gifts. It involves thinking about one's environment and deciding what one will and won't accept.

— MARY PIPHER

There is nothing happens to any person but what was in his power to go through with.

— MARCUS AURELIUS

Difficulty, my brethren, is the nurse of greatness—a harsh nurse, who roughly rocks her foster-children into strength and athletic proportion.

— WILLIAM CULLEN BRYANT

It is odd but agitation or contest of any kind gives a rebound to my spirits and sets me up for a time.

— GEORGE GORDON NOEL BYRON

I have nothing to offer but blood, toil, tears, and sweat.

— WINSTON CHURCHILL

Napoleon said of Massena, that he was not himself until the battle began to go against him; then, when the dead began to fall in ranks around him, awoke his powers of combination, and he put on terror and victory as a robe.

— RALPH WALDO EMERSON

Man needs difficulties; they are necessary for health.

— CARL JUNG

———◆———

Life is truly known only to those who suffer, lose, endure adversity and stumble from defeat to defeat.

— RYSZARD KAPUSCINSKI

———◆———

Do you not see how necessary a world of pains and troubles is to school an intelligence and make it a soul?

— JOHN KEATS

———◆———

I love to see a young girl go out and grab the world by the lapels. Life's a bitch. You've got to go out and kick ass.

— MAYA ANGELOU

———◆———

When among wild beasts, if they menace you, be a wild beast.

— HERMAN MELVILLE

Every time I think I am getting old, and gradually going to the grave, something else happens.

— LILLIAN CARTER

I've been in the twilight of my career longer than most people have had their career.

— MARTINA NAVRATILOVA

We will not be put off the final goal
We have it hidden in us to attain

— ROBERT FROST

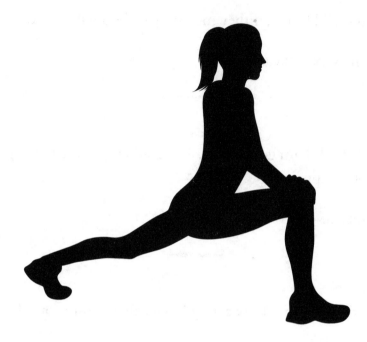

It is day still, you better get busy! Night will intrude when no one can be active.

— JOHANN WOLFGANG VON GOETHE

Nothing is a matter of life and death except life and death.

— ANGELA CARTER

———◆———

Our goal should be to achieve joy.

— ANA CASTILO

———◆———

To be happy is to be able to become aware of oneself without fright.

— WALTER BENJAMIN

———◆———

The aim of life is to live, and to live means to be aware, joyously, drunkenly, serenely, divinely aware.

— HENRY MILLER

———◆———

Awareness requires a rupture with the world we take for granted; then old categories of experience are called into question and revised.

— SHOSHANA ZUBOFF

Humankind has understood history as a series of battles because, to this day, it regards conflict as the central facet of life.

— ANTON CHEKHOV

Here's a victory and defeat—the first and best of victories, the lowest and worst of defeats—which each man gains or sustains at the hands not of another, but of himself.

— PLATO

Not that success, for him, is sure, infallible.
But never has he been afraid to reach.
His lesions are legion.
But reaching is his rule.

— GWENDOLYN BROOKS

People seek a challenge just as fire seeks to flame.

— CHINESE PROVERB

Most people have like plants hidden properties, which chance discloses.

— FRANCOIS DUC DE LA ROCHEFOUCAULD

Courage is a mean with regard to fear and confidence.

— ARISTOTLE

It is a wise man who knows where courage ends and stupidity begins.

— JEROME CADY

Courage is almost a contradiction in terms. It means a strong desire to live taking the form of a readiness to die.

— GILBERT KEITH CHESTERTON

Courage overrides self-doubt, but does not end it.

— MASON COOLEY

Either life entails courage, or it ceases to be life.

— E. M. FORSTER

Courage is only an accumulation of small steps.

— George Konrad

Fortune favors the brave.

— Virgil

Intellectual tasting of life will not supersede muscular activity. If a man should consider the nicety of the passage of a piece of bread down his throat, he would starve.

— Ralph Waldo Emerson

I frequently tramped eight or ten miles through the deepest snow to keep an appointment with a beech tree, or a yellow birch, or an old acquaintance among the pines.

— Henry David Thoreau

Even a runner who is running alone has friends among the squirrels, rocks, snowy egrets, pines, eucalyptus, and wild hay.

— KEVIN NELSON, *THE RUNNER'S BOOK OF DAILY INSPIRATION*

O God, creator of our land. We drink in your creation with our eyes. We listen to the birds' jubilee with our ears.

— ASHANTI PRAYER

Man is never more human than when he plays.

— FRIEDRICH VON SCHILLER

[F]or me, like so many others, running is the answer. Out on the road it is just you, the pavement, and your will.

— JOHN BINGHAM, *THE COURAGE TO START*

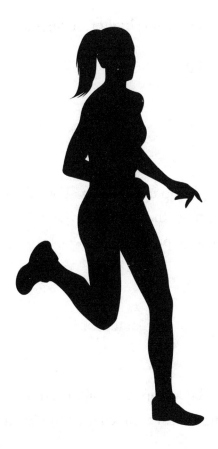

He began to run. Almost immediately he felt easier; felt confidence flow through him as though it were his blood; felt that now, at last, he was in his own country or, more accurately, in his own medium.

— HARRY SYLVESTER, "GOING TO RUN ALL NIGHT"

527

Citius, altius, fortius . . . swifter, higher, stronger.

— OLYMPIC MOTTO

I try not to get too caught up in thinking about the task ahead. I just do what has to be done. I have the belief in myself that what I'm doing is right. Then I let the rest happen.

— EAMONN COGHLAN

There will never be a day when we won't need dedication, discipline, energy, and the feeling that we can change things for the better.

— GEORGE SHEEHAN

To succeed in the marathon at a very high level of competition you have to live in a very stable environment. You need people to support you and help you out. If you don't have this kind of backing, you're not going to make it.

— BILL RODGERS

Keep your dream in front of you. Never let it go regardless of how far-fetched it might seem.

— HAL HIGDON, *MARATHONING A TO Z*

Aside from all the differences that separate us, the magic we share will be the same.

— GRETE WAITZ AND GLORIA AVERBUCH, *RUN YOUR FIRST MARATHON*

Medals are more important than times. Medals stay forever. Times change.

— ROSA MOTA

—◆◈◆—

No one can ever imagine what it's like to stand on the podium and be called one of the world's greatest athletes. What I do in football, I just do it, but nothing will compare to that.

— BOB HAYES, CHAMPION OLYMPIC SPRINTER AND PROFESSIONAL FOOTBALL PLAYER

—◆◈◆—

How do you run a world record? You compress all your baser urges into one minute and forty-two seconds of running.

— PETER COE

—◆◈◆—

Each of us must have a mountain [to climb], even if some might look on it as little more than a hill.

— GEORGE SHEEHAN

The one who believed in themselves the most were the ones who won.

— FLORENCE GRIFFITH JOYNER

The miracle isn't that I finished. . . . The miracle is that I had the courage to start.

— JOHN BINGHAM

Our sporting heroes often strike us as ageless. We remember them in their prime, their faces unblemished, their bodies still taut with power.

— NEAL BASCOMB, *THE PERFECT MILE*

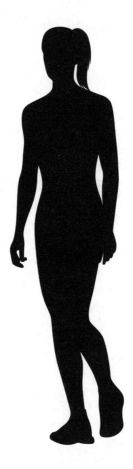

People come out to see you perform and you've got to give them the best you have within you.

— Jesse Owens

The marathon is the stage, and you the performer. The cheers of the crowd are your inspiration.

—GRETE WAITZ AND GLORIA AVERBUCH, *RUN YOUR FIRST MARATHON*

Somebody may beat me, but they are going to have to bleed to do it.

— STEVE PREFONTAINE

You must do the thing you think you cannot do.

— ELEANOR ROOSEVELT

Believe you can do it. Think no other way but "Yes you can." The human body is capable of considerably more physical endurance than most of us realize.

— PAUL REESE

Don't bother just to be better than your contemporaries or predecessors. Try to be better than yourself.

— WILLIAM FAULKNER

———◆———

It's not about how fast you go. It's not about how far you go. It's a process.

— AMBY BURFOOT, *THE RUNNER'S GUIDE TO THE MEANING OF LIFE*

———◆———

Running is my meditation, mind flush, cosmic telephone, mood elevator, and spiritual communion.

— LORRAINE MOLLER

———◆———

In the long run, there will always be family.

— AMBY BURFOOT, *THE RUNNER'S GUIDE TO THE MEANING OF LIFE*

❧

No, but I used to be.

— FRANK SHORTER, WHEN ASKED BY A FAN IF HE WAS FRANK SHORTER

❧

You should learn a lesson from this smaller guy. He was determined and he really tried hard.

— JESSE OWENS TO A GROUP OF YOUNGSTERS, REFERRING TO CARL LEWIS, AT THE JESSE OWENS MEET.

❧

They weren't going to have a party without me.

> — MAURICE GREENE, AFTER SETTING A NEW WORLD RECORD IN THE 200-METER

Track is a hobby, but it is a life too.

> — JIM RYUN

CHAPTER ELEVEN

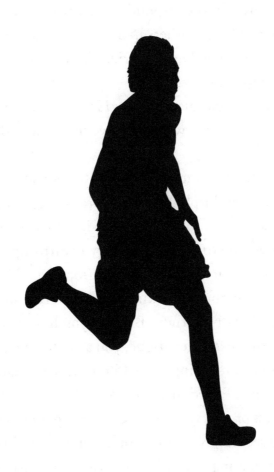

Why runners run

Runner's High

A discussion among participants on my Internet bulletin boards suggested that many of those responding claimed to have experienced the mythical "Runner's High." Others had not. Among the others, I suspect that it was less that they had not experienced the High, but more that they simply failed to recognize it.

Is the High some gargantuan "When Harry Met Sally" orgasm, or is it simply a general feeling of well being we feel now and then when we run?

Scientists have attempted to explain the Runner's High by suggesting that exercise releases endorphins into the brain triggering the emotion, but the evidence seems scanty. I seek less scientific explanations:

If you head down the road without proper warm-up, it may take 10 or 15 minutes to get up to speed in an hour-long run. Then another 10 or 15 minutes to work out all the kinks in your stride so that you are moving smoothly, breathing right. Because you have not yet run far enough to experience extreme fatigue, you start feeling good. And for that third period encompassing 10 or 15 minutes, you encounter what author John Jerome referred to in a book as the "Sweet Spot in Time." Whether at a High or not, you are capable of moving as fast as you can while expending seemingly small amounts of energy. Then fatigue grabs you by the throat, forcing a slowdown during the last 10 or 15 minutes. If you time it right and don't push too hard at the end, you should finish refreshed, feeling a sense of great accomplishment.

Is this the elusive Runner's High? I don't know, but seeking this Sweet Spot is one reason I keep running. I have many reasons. And so does everyone else.

I believe in the runner's high, and I believe that those who are passionate about running are the ones who experience it to the fullest degree possible

— SASHA AZEVEDO

The true but rare runner's high is a zone that we enter when everything seems to click perfectly, when time stands still, and when we can run almost without effort.

— AMBY BURFOOT, *THE RUNNER'S GUIDE TO THE MEANING OF LIFE*

Adrenaline dispels boredom. Run, you sufferers from ennui! Run for your lives!

— MASON COOLEY, *CITY APHORISMS*

Running improves my relationships with my family, my friends, everyone around me. And while my running is personal, it's also something I give. Running can be given.

— TONY SANDOVAL, M.D., WINNER OF THE 1980 U.S. OLYMPIC MARATHON TRIALS

Running became the one event in my daily life that I looked forward to. Books and movies paled in comparison to the refuge of my feet slapping patiently in the fresh morning air.

— KATE KINSEY

He seems to run from within himself.

— EMIL ZATOPEK ON HAILE GEBRSELASSIE

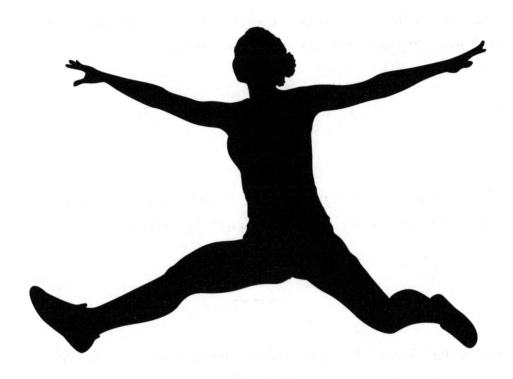

I still bother with runners I call hamburgers. They're never going to run any record times. But they can fulfill their own potential.

— BILL BOWERMAN

541

Happiness is different from pleasure. Happiness has something to do with struggling and enduring and accomplishing.

— GEORGE SHEEHAN

There are clubs you can't belong to, neighborhoods you can't live in, schools you can't get into, but the roads are always open.

— NIKE AD

People don't know why we run, but it's the hard work you put into practice, and the reward you get from the race.

— COURTNEY PARSONS

I run because it's my passion, and not just a sport.

— SASHA AZEVEDO

Life is short. Running makes it seem longer.

— BARON HANSEN

Running was the time he felt most alive. He knew that as surely as he'd ever known anything.

— RICHARD CHRISTIAN MATHESON, "THIRD WIND"

Fitness is a stage you pass through on the way to becoming a runner.

— GEORGE SHEEHAN

Running helps me stay on an even keel and in an optimistic frame of mind.

— BILL CLINTON

My eyes burned with sweat, and I squinted so tight I could hardly see anymore, and because they stung it was impossible to think. I was adjusting, though, lost in rhythm, like a mechanical animal caught on the rim of existence . . . it felt good and I was slipping deep in dreams.

— WALTER McDONALD, "THE TRACK"

It's just simply that I have to.

— EMIL ZATOPEK

It's not a race; it's a state of mind.

— HAL HIGDON, ON THE MARATHON

It's like being on top of the world, and truthfully . . . there's nothing else quite like it!

— SASHA AZEVEDO

The real reason I run is to bring honor to Jesus.

— CHARITY FILLMORE

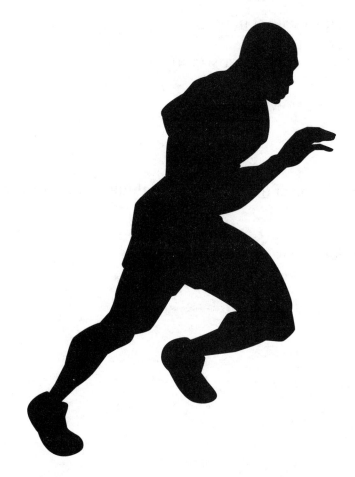

Something in me wanted to find out how far I could run without stopping.

— JACKI HANSON

Running is a great way to relieve stress and clear the mind.

— JOAN VAN ARK

⊶◆⊷

My suspicion is that the effects of running are not extraordinary at all, but quite ordinary. It is the other states, all other feelings, that are peculiar, for they are an abnegation of the way you and I are supposed to feel. As runners, I think we reach directly back along the endless chain of history.

— JAMES W. FIXX, *THE COMPLETE BOOK OF RUNNING*

⊶◆⊷

Sometimes I'll have a problem while working on a piece and I'll say, "Wait a second, I need a break." I get our spaniel, Thunder, head out for a run, and 50 minutes later, when I try the passage again, it's easy. Running clears the head.

— MISHA DICHTER, CLASSICAL PIANIST

I am not sure that I can describe what has been called the "runner's high," but like poetry and beauty, I know it when I experience it.

— MATTHEW SHAFNER

My feelings tried to control me on my run. I had to concentrate fully on forthcoming running and success. I wanted to triumph.

— CATHY FREEMAN

You have to wonder at times what you're doing out there. Over the years, I've given myself a thousand reasons to keep running, but it always comes back to where it started. It comes down to self-satisfaction and a sense of achievement.

— STEVE PREFONTAINE

I can't imagine living and not running.

— PAULA RADCLIFFE

It is the athlete's job to learn to do the hard things easily.

— JOHN JEROME, *THE SWEET SPOT IN TIME*

My times become slower and slower, but the experience of the race is unchanged: each race a drama, each race a challenge, each race stretching me in one way or another, and each race telling me more about myself and others.

— GEORGE SHEEHAN

I do a lot of running and hiking, and I also collect stamps.

— SALLY RIDE

I always have loved running, since I was fifteen.

— BILL RODGERS

I loved the feeling of freedom in running, the fresh air, the feeling that the only person I'm competing with is me.

— WILMA RUDOLPH

I enjoy the freedom of running and the challenge of training and competition as much now as when I first started back in high school.

— ALBERTO SALAZAR

Handball, swimming, running, jumping, basketball, and boxing were as much a part of me as breathing.

— GENE TUNNEY

A lot of people run a race to see who is fastest. I run to see who has the most guts, who can punish himself into exhausting pace, and then at the end, punish himself even more.

— STEVE PREFONTAINE

When [the runner's high] does set in, usually around three or four miles, my body flows into a smooth rhythm and my mind is no longer conscious of how far or how long I've run or how much farther to go.

— MATTHEW SHAFNER

For me, running is a lifestyle and an art. I'm more interested in the magic of it than the mechanics.

— LORRAINE MOLLER

My running was very simple; it was out of myself. Perhaps sometimes I was like a mad dog. It didn't matter about style or what it looked like to others; there were records to break.

— EMIL ZATOPEK

To me, the runner's high is a sensational reaction to a great run! It's an exhilarating feeling of satisfaction and achievement.

— SASHA AZEVEDO

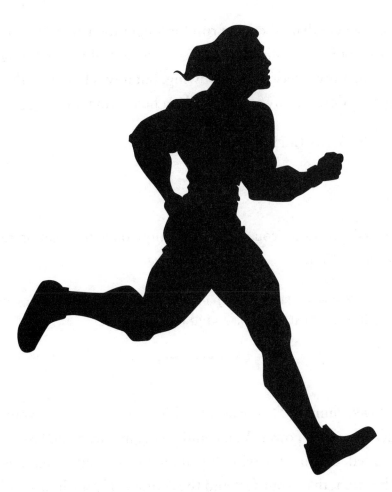

There are as many reasons for running as there are days in the year, years in my life. But mostly I run because I am an animal and a child, an artist and a saint. So, too, are you. Find your own play, your own self-renewing compulsion, and you will become the person you are meant to be.

— GEORGE SHEEHAN

I read somewhere that when you run for longer than an hour, your body begins to adapt in miraculous ways. I couldn't actually have thought, even then, that my arteries were growing, but it was like that. I'd go for a 20 and glance down at my sternum, like a hen sitting on an egg.

— BENJAMIN CHEEVER, *STRIDES*

Mr. Rodgers, why don't you concentrate more on your vocation rather than your avocation.

— THE SCHOOL PRINCIPAL, TO BILL RODGERS, AT THE SCHOOL WHERE RODGERS TAUGHT FOR A LIVING

I always loved running . . . it was something you could do by yourself, and under your own power. You could go in any direction, fast or slow as you wanted, fighting the wind if you felt like it, seeking out new sights just on the strength of your feet and the courage of your lungs.

— JESSE OWENS

If one could run without getting tired, I don't think one would often want to do anything else.

— C.S. Lewis

———◆———

I feel the earth and the wind and the trees. I feel its spirit. It puts me in the moment. I feel the rhythm of the race. It's like music. When the rhythm gets dissonant and chaotic, it is either a jazzy driving force behind me or demons inside me.

— Gabriel Jennings

———◆———

Everyone wants beautiful legs.

— Peter Martins and New York City Ballet, *New York City Ballet Workout*

———◆———

There is no such thing as an average runner. We are all above average.

— HAL HIGDON, *MARATHONING A TO Z*

I didn't want to run Boston to prove anything. I just fell in love with the marathon.

— ROBERTA GIBB ON RUNNING THE BOSTON MARATHON

I like running because it's a challenge. If you run hard, there's the pain— and you've got to work your way through the pain. You know, lately it seems all you hear is "Don't overdo it" and "Don't push yourself." Well, I think that's a lot of bull. If you push the human body, it will respond.

— BOB CLARKE, PHILADELPHIA FLYERS GENERAL MANAGER, NHL HALL OF FAME.

I always ran through fear—of being beaten. It brought out the best in me, being terrified of being beaten.

— SHIRLEY STRICKLAND DE LA HUNTY

CHAPTER TWELVE

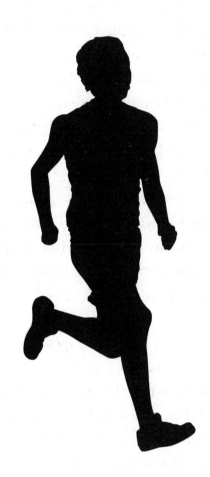

Witty running commentary

A Funny Thing Happened on the Way to the Finish Line

We runners are a motley bunch. Consider how we dress, specifically before a marathon. Given our high demographics, we should look like bankers and fashion models wearing Pradas and Brooks Brother suits, but we arrive at the Expo one notch above the Homeless.

Muddied running shoes. Faded jeans. Aged T-shirt from one race. Billed cap from another. Nylon jacket from a third. The highest fashion statement we can make is that we acquired that jacket at the Boston Marathon, 100th running in 1996, meaning it has been thrown in the washer one hundred times.

But we are the chosen people, who arrive at the starting line dressed in upside-down garbage bags carrying bottles with yellowed liquid: Gatorade before we drink, urine afterwards. During the course of our 26-mile-385-yard journeys, we acquire: a) bloody nipples, b) black toes and c) so much salt clinging to our bodies that it appears we just took a swim in the Dead Sea.

And as we stagger through the streets, spectators shout from the sidelines, "You're looking good!"

Once finished, we collapse into the arms of some stranger who wraps around our sunburned shoulders a Mylar blanket that crinkles as we walk and displays the name of some bank, shoe company or department store. We have just paid $100 to enter this race, and now we have to spend the rest of the day looking like an aluminum billboard. And even if we have not barfed up that Gatorade, you do not want to kiss us.

The next day, however, we do look good: with that finisher's medal hung around our shoulders.

Running is like mouthwash; if you can feel the burn, it's working.

— BRIAN TACKETT

———⋙◆⋘———

My most vivid memories of beginning to run are of how little anyone seemed to know about the sport and how little was available in way of information and equipment. . .when I went to a newsstand to try to find a running magazine, it was hopeless. "Running," I told the vendor, who looked quite puzzled. "You know—track and field." His eyes lit up in seeming recognition. Then he handed me *Road & Track*, a magazine about cars.

— FRED LEBOW

———⋙◆⋘———

I'll get up in the morning while they've all got hangovers and run my five miles. But the women who do run are usually ten years younger than me and they're really obsessed about running. That's all they do. They're really boring.

— TRISHA GODDARD

———⋙◆⋘———

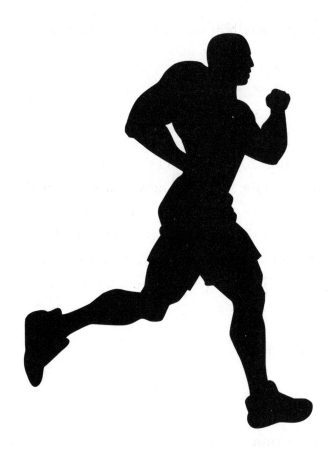

All that running and exercise can do for you is make you healthy.

— DENNY MCCLAIN

Before he rounds the brushy curves, we see him, his French running shoes, his shorts, his naked legs, his T-shirt advertising something unimaginable, his terry sweatband, his tiny nylon wallet fastened to his shoe ingeniously with Velcro—who once was never seen without a coat and necktie—hairy wool, rumpled linen, bleached-to-the-bone starched cotton broadcloth, stained shimmering reptilian silk—who hated zippers as much as polyester, snaps as much as leisure suits.

> — Lon Otto, "We Cannot Save Him"

The pleasure of jogging and running is rather like that of wearing a fur coat in Texas in August: the true joy comes in being able to take the damn thing off.

> — Joseph Epstein

If you come to think of it, you never see deer, dogs, and rabbits worrying about their menus, and yet they run much faster than humans.

> — Emil Zatopek

Even in high school, you were some kind of fruitcake if you ran, like you were naked in the wind. Nobody else did it; there were no cheerleaders or anything like that.

— CHARLIE RODGERS

Lady, you just passed it.

— SPECTATOR TO JOAN BENOIT SAMUELSON, WHEN SHE ASKED IN THE 1979 BOSTON MARATHON HOW FAR AWAY HEARTBREAK HILL WAS

Dick Cheney said he was running again. He said his health was fine. "I've got a doctor with me twenty-four hours a day." Yeah, that's always the sign of a man in good health, isn't it?

— DAVID LETTERMAN

I love going somewhere where somebody is mouthing off about how much money he makes or how important he is, and I don't say anything, but inside I'm thinking, "The only thing that's in shape on him is his mouth."

— DOUG MOCK

<hr/>

The man who has made the mile record is W. G. George. . . . His time was 4 minutes 12.75 seconds and the probability is that his record will never be beaten.

— HARRY ANDREWS IN 1903

<hr/>

It's the road signs, 'Beware of lions.'

— KIP LAGAT, KENYAN DISTANCE RUNNER, DURING THE SYDNEY OLYMPICS, EXPLAINING WHY HIS COUNTRY PRODUCES SO MANY GREAT RUNNERS

Runner's high? Isn't that where two runners pass in the park and one says, "Hi." And the other returns the greeting?

— HAL HIGDON

I signed up for track in high school as it was the easiest team to join; no cuts and everyone is guaranteed a position.

— KIM AHRENS

Sweat cleanses from the inside. It comes from places a shower will never reach.

— GEORGE SHEEHAN

I've never seen a computer jogging.

> — BASKETBALL COACH FRANK LAYDEN ON WHY COMPUTERS ARE
> SMARTER THAN PEOPLE

Hell, no. When I die I want to be sick.

> — ABE LEMONS WHEN ASKED IF HE RUNS

I guess the difference is that running makes me feel good, and the other stuff makes me feel bad.

> — DON IMUS ON BEING ADDICTED TO RUNNING VERSUS BEING ADDICTED
> TO SMOKING AND DRINKING

I learned not to take the lead if I wasn't sure where the finish line was.

> — PAT PETERSEN, WHO GOT LOST IN HIS FIRST HIGH-SCHOOL CROSS
> COUNTRY RACE

After the first six-mile loop, Harry Murphy . . . offered me a cup of whisky. I gulped it down . . . After the next six-mile loop, I happily downed another cup of whisky. On the third loop, someone gave me a cup of water. I was so disappointed!

— FRED LEBOW ON HIS EXPERIENCE AT THE CHERRY TREE MARATHON IN THE BRONX IN 1970

"A sunny day in winter" is a nice way of describing the seasoned runner. I've heard worse.

— ROGER ROBINSON

When I jog I joggle.

— OGDEN NASH

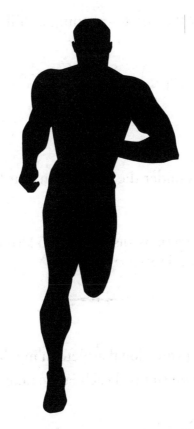

A man who sets out to become an artist at the mile is something like a man who sets out to discover the most graceful method of being hanged. No matter how logical his plans, he cannot carry them out without physical suffering.

— PAUL O'NEIL, *SPORTS ILLUSTRATED*, MAY 31, 1956

Two things are bad for the heart—running uphill and running down people.

— BERNARD GIMBEL

I am quite sure she was under the impression that I had run four miles in one minute.

— ROGER BANNISTER ON HIS GIRLFRIEND MOYRA JACOBSSON'S LACK OF INTEREST IN HIS RUNNING

Distance-running, to a professional athlete in my day, was five laps around the field. And you stopped each lap to take your pulse.

— LYNN SWANN

While running, it is rude to count the people you pass out loud.

— ANONYMOUS

Even if you fall flat on your face at least you are moving forward.

— SUE LUKE

———◆·◆———

Maybe I shouldn't have had breakfast at Denny's.

— JORDAN KENT, WHO VOMITED AFTER RUNNING THE 400 METERS
IN THE 2002 USA JUNIOR NATIONAL CHAMPIONSHIPS HELD IN
EUGENE, OR

———◆·◆———

Running on worn-out shoes is like driving on bald tires. You might make the next town, but then again, you might have a blow out.

— RUNNING SHOP OWNER

———◆·◆———

In the very first race in literature, the old guy wins. He's Odysseus (AKA Ulysses), pushing forty at the time, and he beats the best of the united Greek army gathered outside Troy.

— ROGER ROBINSON

———◆·◆———

The course reads like a wine list. Chateau Beychevelle, Chateau Gruaud-Larose, and Chateau Lafite Rothschild all ornament the route and all provide libations. The motto: "Médoc, le Marathon le Plus Long du Monde." The T-shirt pictures a drunken runner staggering through a vineyard.

— BENJAMIN CHEEVER ON THE MÉDOC MARATHON IN *STRIDES*

The trouble with jogging is that the ice falls out of your glass.

— MARTIN MULL

[I]t's nice to be 40—at least I usually win my age group!

— FRANCIE LARRIEU SMITH

We can't all be heroes because someone has to sit on the curb and clap as they go by.

> — WILL ROGERS

I'm going to go out a winner if I have to find a high school race to win my last race.

> — JOHNNY GRAY

Finland has produced so many brilliant distance runners because back home it costs $2.50 a gallon for gas.

> — ESA TIKKANNEN IN 1979

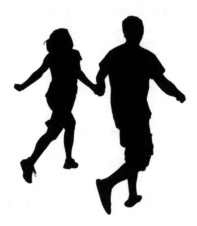

I think it is bloody silly to put flowers on the grave of the 4-minute mile, now isn't it? It turns out it wasn't so much like Everest as it was like the Matterhorn; somebody had to climb it first, but I hear now they've even got a cow up it.

— HARRY WILSON

When I turned 40, there were no more good shoes.

— *BILL RODGERS' LIFETIME RUNNING PLAN*

[R]unning in a pretty muddy cross country race, one of my shoes stuck in the mud and came off. . . . I really got aggressive with myself, and [started] to pass a lot of runners. . . . I improved something like twenty places. . . . But I never did get my shoe back.

— ROB DE CASTELLA

If you grunt, grimace, grind, and pound your way through a run and then you limp home 15 minutes later, you may want to consider changing your style.

— *RUNNING FOR DUMMIES*

Kids can watch [other sports] start to finish, in real time. . . . But the men's 400 relay finals at the world championships? On your mark, get set . . . we'll show it to you in four hours on another network.

— MIKE PENNER, "TRACK AND FIELD, TV HAS A PROBLEM WITH YOU," *LOS ANGELES TIMES*, AUGUST 13, 2001

I said running a sub-2:20 would be a cakewalk after this.

— JOAN BENOIT SAMUELSON ON GIVING BIRTH TO HER DAUGHTER

A critic is a legless man who teaches running.

— CHANNING POLLOCK

If the hill has its own name, then it's probably a pretty tough hill.

— MARTY STERN

Only one hill today, boys.

— JOCK SEMPLE, AT THE START OF THE MOUNT WASHINGTON ROAD RACE

The first time I see a jogger smiling, I'll consider it.

— JOAN RIVERS

———◦———

Have you ever noticed? Anyone going slower than you is an idiot, and anyone going faster than you is a maniac?

— GEORGE CARLIN

———◦———

I will even try eating worms and caterpillar fungus. It might improve my jogging, and for sure it will improve my flossing.

— SCOTT OSTLER IN THE *SAN FRANCISCO CHRONICLE*

———◦———

There ain't no shame looking at a good runner's back. Now, if the runner sucks, that's something else entirely. . .

— THE RAGE, TRAINING TIPS, "COMEBACK"

———◦———

The event that certainly tries men's soles.

— JERRY NASON ON THE BOSTON MARATHON, IN 1945

If you are noticing the scenery, you probably aren't working hard.

— SEBASTIAN COE

If you run every day until you're 90 years old, I guarantee that you'll live a long life.

— *BILL RODGERS' LIFETIME RUNNING PLAN*

There are actually people who cheat at race walks [. . .]. You know you've given up in life when you cheat at a race walk. You've decided that you're so pathetic the only way you can win is by cheating against people who aren't even competing.

— MICHAEL LOGSDON

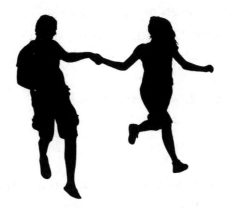

[I]f I listened to my body, I'd live on toffee pops and port wine.

— ROGER ROBINSON

—◆—

Start slow, then taper off.

— WALT STACK

—◆—

If you ask my younger daughter what I do, she'll tell you that I'm the fastest runner in the world. In other words, she doesn't know much about running.

— *BILL RODGERS' LIFETIME RUNNING PLAN*

If you want to know what you'll look like in ten years, look in the mirror after you've run a marathon.

— JEFF SCAFF

Hills: You entered a marathon with hills? You idiot.

— DON KARDONG'S MARATHON ADVICE

Who runs in circles never gets far.

— THORNTON W. BURGESS, BOWSER THE HOUND

Running won't kill you, you'll pass out first!

— ANONYMOUS

———◆———

[W]hen I go to competitions the young girls don't look upon me as a granny. Except if you are Uta Pippig. One day I was out training, and she said to me, "Heh, Cilla, you could be my mother."

— PRISCILLA WELCH

———◆———

I go running when I have to. When the ice cream truck is doing sixty.

— WENDY LIEBMAN

———◆———

I have been passed in races by tall runners and short runners. I have been passed by runners who look as though they have not eaten in six weeks, and by runners who appear to have just wiped out an all-you-can-eat breakfast bar.

— JOHN BINGHAM, *THE COURAGE TO START*

The primary reason to have a coach is to have somebody who can look at you and say, "Man, you're looking good today."

— JACK DANIELS

Jogging is very beneficial. It's good for your legs and your feet. It's also very good for the ground. It makes it feel needed.

— CHARLES SCHULZ, *PEANUTS*

When runners win a big race these days, they get a car. When I won a big race, I got a ride.

— RON DELANY

To a runner, a side stitch is like a car alarm. It signifies something is wrong, but you ignore it until it goes away.

— ANONYMOUS

It's unnatural for people to run around the city streets unless they are thieves or victims. It makes people nervous to see someone running. I know that when I see someone running on my street, my instincts tell me to let the dog go after him.

— MIKE ROYKO

I don't generally like running. I believe in training by rising gently up and down from the bench.

— SATCHEL PAIGE

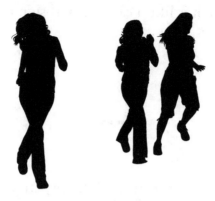

School cross country runs started because the rugby pitches were flooded. There was an alternative: extra studying. This meant there were plenty of runners on sports afternoons.

— GORDON PIRIE

I believe that the Good Lord gave us a finite number of heartbeats and I'm damned if I'm going to use up mine running up and down a street.

— NEIL ARMSTRONG

I don't think jogging is healthy, especially morning jogging. If morning joggers knew how tempting they looked to morning motorists, they would stay home and do sit-ups.

— RITA RUDNER

Runners just do it—they run for the finish line even if someone else has reached it first.

— ANONYMOUS

"Why aren't you signed up for the 401K?"
"I'd never be able to run that far."

— SCOTT ADAMS, *DILBERT* (4/2/01)

Avoid any diet that discourages the use of hot fudge.

— DON KARDONG

Sex before the race? Fine, it will do you no harm. But try not to distract the starter.

— ROGER ROBINSON

The only reason I would take up jogging is so that I could hear heavy breathing again.

— ERMA BOMBECK

Exercise is done against one's wishes and maintained only because the alternative is worse.

— GEORGE SHEEHAN

My doctor recently told me that jogging could add years to my life. I think he was right. I feel ten years older already.

— MILTON BERLE

The cup spills if I run.

— BILL RODGERS WHEN ASKED WHY HE STOPPED TO TAKE WATER BREAKS DURING THE BOSTON MARATHON. HE SET A RECORD IN THAT RACE.

I was looking for God during the last mile, but I didn't see Him. I guess He finished ahead of me too.

— ALBERT MABUS, LAST MALE FINISHER AT THE 2001 NITTANY VALLEY HALF MARATHON

I get my exercise running to the funerals of my friends who exercise.

— BARRY GRAY

———◆———

Technically, these guys did not run entirely from coast to coast contiguously, because they crossed the Hudson River and Mississippi River by ferry.

— PAUL REESE, CROSS USA RUNNER, WHO COVERED BOTH RIVERS BY
RUNNING ACROSS BRIDGES, SPEAKING OF EARLIER RUNNERS.

———◆———

Most of the top runners I know feel the same way about diet. They're skeptical about nutrition being the prime element in racing success, but they like to check each other's grocery lists. Just in case.

— DON KARDONG

———◆———

I am not ashamed to say that I don't like to *run* anywhere, unless it's really extremely urgent, like if I pull into the Denny's parking lot at 4:59, knowing the Senior Dinner Discount stops at 5:00. Also, I've recently discovered that when I run anywhere at my age, my belly button arrives at my destination about three minutes before I do.

— MICHAEL MILLIGAN, *GRANDPA RULES*

Practice doesn't make perfect. Perfect practice makes perfect.

— PETER MARTINS AND NEW YORK CITY BALLET, *NEW YORK CITY BALLET WORKOUT*

Running is the best anti-depressant on the market, with virtually no cost or negative side effects.

— HAL HIGDON, *MARATHONING A TO Z*

CHAPTER THIRTEEN

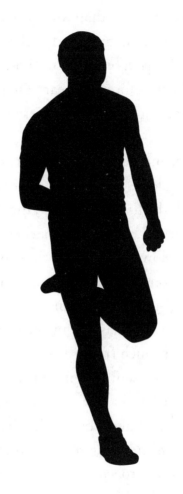

Our "Gigantic" running miscellany

Running with the Pack, Part II

Is there a lovelier piece of music than Mozart's 21st piano concerto, the C-Major? The second movement served as the theme song for the 1967 Swedish film, *Elvira Madigan*, but most of those running marathons today were not even born before that year. They train wearing iPods tuned to electronic beats, not subtle melodies written by some eighteenth century composer.

I don't own an iPod, and despite my love of Mozart, I concede that his 21st piano concerto would be a poor choice for working out. You'd get off to a good start with the first movement, the *Allegro* (or fast), but then you collide with the second movement, marked *Andante*, a word that tells the orchestra to play it slowly. It would bring you to a halt as a runner. Even the tumultuous Rondo in the third and final movement, another *Allegro*, might not get you moving again.

Nevertheless, the waters of classical music run deep, not shallow. As runners, we can learn as much from the format in which the music is written as from the music itself. When I write training programs for runners, I usually prescribe a hard day to push the muscles, followed by an easy day to rest them, followed by another hard day to build on what went before. *Allegro, Andante, Allegro.* Oregon coach Bill Bowerman pioneered the hard/easy approach.

Mozart knew how to blend fast and slow movements just as Bowerman knew how to blend fast and slow workouts.

It may be a stretch to suggest that Mozart can teach us how to train for road races. Maybe it is enough merely to enjoy his music, still popular today even on some iPods, then run to your own beat.

I have to train him not only to represent Michigan. I have to train him to represent the United States.

— RON WARHURST ON ALAN WEBB

Every time I have a personal or work problem, I go for a run.

— FRED LEBOW

Every day is a good day when you run.

— KEVIN NELSON, *THE RUNNER'S BOOK OF DAILY INSPIRATION*

You start pounding out a couple dozen 5- or 6-minute miles and you start to feel such a sense of satisfaction and peace you can't believe it. Sure you're tired, and sure you're sore, but if you could bottle the high you get from transcending the pain mile after mile after mile, well . . . reality was overrated.

— DICK BEARDSLEY

Running made us human, at least in an anatomical sense.

— DR. DANIEL E. LIEBERMAN

It was a carnival of pain, but he loved each stride because the running distilled him to essence and the heat hastened this distillation.

— JAMES TABOR, "THE RUNNER"

I don't know when I made the transformation from running as a sport to running as part of my life. I can't separate the two.

— GAIL W. KISLEVITZ

We are here to be heroes. The marathon is the one way we prove it to ourselves.

— GEORGE SHEEHAN

I just decided I was going to run the race. It wasn't for prize money. I didn't even realize at that point women weren't allowed to run.

— BOBBI GIBB ON THE BOSTON MARATHON

—◆—

Elvis Costello once said, "Writing about music is like dancing about architecture." In the same way, running—the total, exalted, painful, glorious, miserable, purifying, filthy, rhythmic, dream, transcendent, achy experience—for the most part defies rendition in words.

— GARTH BATTISTA

—◆—

Runners are also the type who have been known to meticulously polish and shine their treadmills every three days and religiously wax the revolving belt, but the last oil change and wash for their car occurred some 40,000 miles ago.

— BOB SCHWARTZ, *I RUN, THEREFORE I AM—NUTS*

—◆—

I guess I tend to choose individual sports like swimming, running, or ocean sailing because I have to rely on myself.

— RICK BACHMANN

I believe that by living as athletes we live more fully.

— GLORIA AVERBUCH

Are you truly dirty if you don't take a shower every day? No, but you feel that way. It's the same with running. Just like a shower, running is part of my daily life.

— NINA KUSCSIK

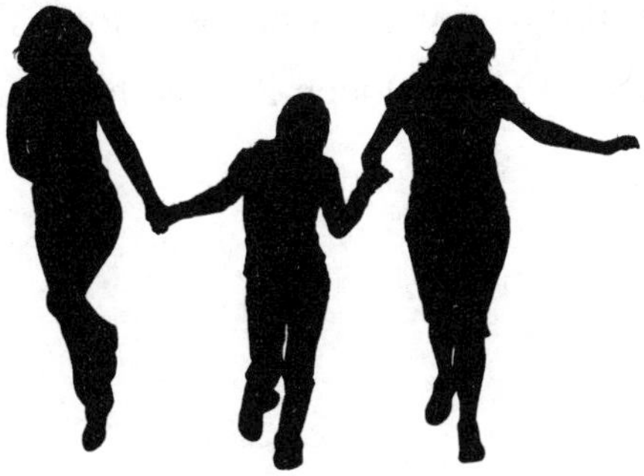

The pain I experienced in the marathon wasn't the type where I felt a sense of helplessness, like being in a car accident. I had control over the pain, could have stopped it if I chose to.

— BILL BEGG

Deep down I always believe I can win.

— FRANCIE LARRIEU SMITH

At twenty miles I wanted to cry. . . . I needed nourishment in the worst way and then I spotted a Dairy Queen across the street. Soft ice cream, the perfect food!

— RICHARD BELLICCHI

There is something about running that knocks down the "Berlin Walls" of race, religion, custom, and language that divide us, reminding us—as Alberto Juantorena says—that we all have "not four eyes, but two."

— MICHAEL SANDROCK

I didn't just want to run, I wanted to run as far and as fast as I could, as was humanly possible.

— TED CORBITT

I read in the sports section about Roger Bannister breaking the four-minute mile. I couldn't comprehend the speed of a four-minute mile, so I got on my bike, rode to Wingate Field which had a track, climbed over the three-tier cyclone fence, and ran around the track once as fast as I could and timed myself at 1:25.

— NINA KUSCSIK

———◆———

I do think there are lots of kids out there who have the potential to be great runners if only they have the right coach, someone who shows an interest and cares.

— BILL RODGERS

———◆———

When I took my artificial right leg for a 26.2-mile run in 1976, I had no idea how it would change my life. I entered the New York City Marathon that year because I was a runner and that is what runners do.

— DICK TRAUM

———◆———

I never was a good track runner; psychologically, the laps killed me.

— KATHRINE SWITZER

⸺◆⸺

This is not about instant gratification. You have to work hard for it, sweat for it, give up sleeping in on Sunday mornings.

— LAUREN FESSENDEN

⸺◆⸺

The input is considerable but the rewards are unbelievable.

— ROB HEMMEL

⸺◆⸺

Running changed my life and brought it into balance. I now feel as though my entire essence, body, and soul is centered.

— DONNA ISAACSON

⸺◆⸺

There's nothing quite like your first marathon. The adrenaline just flows.

— SISTER MARION IRVINE

It didn't matter that we were last. We knew we were finishing, that we would endure to the end.

— THOMAS KING

I died at twenty miles. I was tired and thought, I will never do this again. This is crazy. Even Kenyans get tired after running that far.

— PAUL MBUGUA

Stopping is an honorable tradition in running.

— KEVIN NELSON, *THE RUNNER'S BOOK OF DAILY INSPIRATION*

The thing I worried about most was courage. Would I have the courage to keep running if it really hurt, if it got harder than I was used to, if Heartbreak Hill broke me?

— KATHRINE SWITZER

Wes Santee . . . John Landy . . . Roger Bannister . . . Who is going to be the first to reach the end of the rainbow and run the fabled four-minute mile?

— THE ASSOCIATED PRESS IN 1953

The world obviously would like to see a 4:00 mile, but let's keep it kosher in a regularly fixed race.

— JESSE ABRAMSON IN THE *NEW YORK HERALD TRIBUNE*

The steady encroachment of commerce into modern athletics over the years has taken some of the romance out of the mile record.

— NEAL BASCOMB

———✦———

There is no formula for how many wins, records, or medals a runner must earn to qualify as "a legend." Rather, the sobriquet is reserved for those who carry a mystique that transcends the finish line, making them much more than champion athletes.

— MICHAEL SANDROCK

———✦———

It is tempting to extrapolate athletic records to the future and assume they will improve forever. The obvious, trivial truth is, they won't.

— BERND HEINRICH, *WHY WE RUN: A NATURAL HISTORY*

———✦———

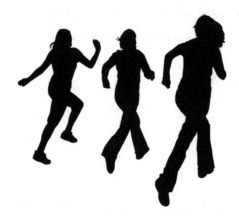

I know I can run a marathon, ironically something I couldn't do in my younger years. This aging thing isn't so bad after all.

— JIM MILLER

I had no interest in finishing. My only thought was how to get home.

— BILL RODGERS ON HIS FIRST MARATHON

In Kenmore Square stood the baseball immortal Ted Williams. He was clapping with admiration for all who passed. A friend of mine actually heard him say, "Now *those* are real athletes."

— ERICH SEGAL ON HIS FIRST BOSTON MARATHON

Post-race refreshments serve as the catalyst for seeing how many bananas and bagels we can consume in the span of our best 800-meter time. We often burn more calories racing around the refreshment tables than we do during the run itself.

— BOB SCHWARTZ, *I RUN, THEREFORE I AM—NUTS*

No other amputee had attempted to run a marathon before. The norms of society, and of sport, dictated that it was an impossible event, but I was soon to let it be known that it was, indeed, possible.

— DICK TRAUM

This was definitely harder than any track course I had run. . . . I didn't like this marathon racing.

— GRETE WAITZ ON HER FIRST MARATHON

——◆——

It was a whole different game once we got to the hills. We had been running really slow, and from my point of view that was fine. But once we started up, he began pushing the pace at an intensity that neither of us could continue to the finish. It was only a matter of time before either he would break me, or he would have to slow down himself.

— ALBERTO SALAZAR ON THE COMPETITION BETWEEN HIM AND DICK BEARDSLEY AT THE 1982 BOSTON MARATHON

——◆——

[W]omen like Olympian Paula Radcliffe have world record marathon times that are sub-2:20—that's more than two hours faster than the first woman known to run a marathon in 1896.

— SHANTI SOSIENSKI, *WOMEN WHO RUN*

——◆——

Nothing hurts more, but is so rewarding at the same time.

— SANDY ZANCHI ON THE MARATHON

—⟛◆⟚—

What if this were your only chance? Sure, it'll be painful, but what's pain?

— FRANZ STAMPFL

—⟛◆⟚—

Do you not know that in a race all the runners run, but only one gets the prize. Run in such a way as to get the prize.

— ST. PAUL, CORINTHIANS 9:24

—⟛◆⟚—

We all need goals. Life is hard to live without one.

— TORY BAUCUM

—⟛◆⟚—

[Running] pervades my life. I wouldn't go so far as to say it has crept into other parts of my life; I would rather say it has become its own part of my life.

— LARRY SMITH

[Running] is my private time, my therapy, my religion.

— GAIL W. KISLEVITZ

The combined feeling of exhaustion, euphoria, and accomplishment is quite luxurious.

— LARRY SMITH ON HOW IT FEELS AFTER FINISHING A MARATHON

On a good day, it all blends. I feel a part of a private universe where everything comes together and feels great.

— MATTHEW SHAFNER

I had to learn how to drink while running. That sounds easy, but it's like rubbing your head and patting your stomach at the same time.

— KIM AHRENS

I couldn't fail, as no other amputee had ever attempted to run a marathon before.

— DICK TRAUM

I definitely think the high school coaches should take the opportunity to educate runners that this is a sport that will take them through life.

— KIM AHRENS

I learned quickly that if I had to talk to Coach on the phone, I'd better do it early in the day. If I talked to him at, say, eight o'clock at night, I couldn't get to sleep. I wanted to run the workout right then. He'd get me so fired up I'd just lie in bed feeling the adrenaline pound its way through my body.

— DICK BEARDSLEY ON BILL SQUIRES

Haile always wants to please everyone. For example, the Ethiopian people want to see Haile Gebrselassie win, so he keeps running even though he has won everything there is to win. And when he loses, he's not necessarily upset because he didn't achieve something he wanted, but because he didn't achieve what others wanted.

— GETANEH RETA ON HAILE GEBRSELASSIE

I went at each race like there was a gold medal at stake. It wasn't like I ran one hard, then slacked off the next. Every time it was my best effort. I didn't know how to go at it any other way.

— DICK BEARDSLEY

That was the first time I had seen runners at close quarters. They appeared as normal human beings, not demigods as I had imagined.

— KENYAN RUNNER PAUL TERGAT ON SEEING RUNNERS AT THE ALL-AFRICAN GAMES AS A CHILD

⎯⊷◆⊶⎯

Pasta (despite some recent attacks that question just how much nutritional punch the noodle wields) has traditionally been the darling of the pre-race meal.

— MARK WILL-WEBER

⎯⊷◆⊶⎯

He took in even, deep measures of cool air with mechanical regularity, disinterestedly feeling inside his chest the huge heart muscle thumping its slow liquid drumbeat.

— JOHN L. PARKER JR., *ONCE A RUNNER*

[A]t age forty-three, when I found myself standing in my garage in a new pair of running shoes, I knew that it was my moment of truth . . . Behind me lay forty years of bad decisions and broken promises.

— JOHN BINGHAM, *THE COURAGE TO START*

———◆———

Running is a kind of investment in yourself.

— *THE RUNNER'S BOOK OF DAILY INSPIRATION*, KEVIN NELSON

———◆———

It has been said that the love of the chase is an inherent delight in man— a relic of an instinctive passion.

— CHARLES DARWIN

———◆———

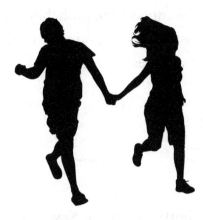

The fastest human can run about 10 meters a second for about 10 seconds. Your typical squirrel can double that for 4 or 5 minutes.

— Dr. Daniel E. Lieberman

—◆—

Today, [endurance running] is primarily a form of exercise and recreation, but its roots may be as ancient as the origin of the human genus, and its demands a major contributing factor to the human body form.

—*Nature*

—◆—

[S]everal important truths support the probability that we became big-game hunters by chasing animals, our potential victims getting larger as we modified our bodies for speed.

— ELIZABETH MARSHALL THOMAS IN *THE OLD WAY: A STORY OF THE FIRST PEOPLE*

I pull on my extralong shorts, tie up my New Balance 991s, run past the barricades and blast walls that surround the compound where I live, and slip into Baghdad's anarchic streets.

— *NEW YORK TIMES* CORRESPONDENT DEXTER FILKINS IN *RUNNER'S WORLD*

[Running] makes a wide variety of people palatable to each other. This seems to be true of all serious endeavors.

— BENJAMIN CHEEVER, *STRIDES*

We have a magnificent motor at our disposal, but we no longer know how to use it.

— EMIL ZATOPEK

I know what it feels like when I'm running great. And when I'm off, I want to know why.

— FRANCIE LARRIEU SMITH

Sharp runs so that the body may be emptied of moisture.

— HIPPOCRATES'S RECOMMENDATION

When they're out there running, for that little slice of time, they're not free, but they have a little bit of mental release.

> — LAURA BOWMAN, WHO IS IN CHARGE OF A RUNNING CLUB FOR PRISONERS

It is a belief that finds no support in other fields of endeavor. The child learning to write, the pianist who practices for six hours a day, the bricklayer laying bricks—the work of these people does not deteriorate as a result of constant repetition of the same movements.

> — FRANZ STAMPFL, DENYING THE BELIEF THAT OVERTRAINING LEADS TO WORSE PERFORMANCE

The racers of antiquity who purposed competing at the Olympic games were extremely careful that nothing should interfere with the rapidity of their pace; and with this object, they paid special attention to the condition of their spleen, believing that the unhealthy condition of that organ renders the whole body heavy and the breath short.

— CHARLES RUSSELL, *WONDERS OF BODILY STRENGTH AND SKILL IN ALL AGES AND ALL COUNTRIES*

Coupling good writing with good running is an extraordinarily difficult task, as the sport is innately interior, and impossibly complex.

— GARTH BATTISTA

The boy's face was ash-pale and his lips, wrenched back from his teeth, were white. He was cotton-mouthed, racking for breath, but he was keeping his chin down. He was pulling with his arms. He was making every stride laboriously, in an agony of willpower. But he was making it. He was running.

— EDDY ORCUTT, "WHEELBARROW"

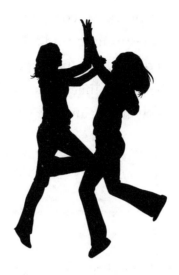

Often the very act of starting a race was seen as a protest.

— CHARLOTTE LETTIS RICHARDSON

❦

[L]egendary athletes are perhaps at the top of running's pyramid, but it is the common runners who make up its base and who are the foundation of our sport.

— MICHAEL SANDROCK

❦

Running clubs are great places. In England, the running club is the hub of your whole social life. It's the hub of your whole damn life.

— DAVE WELCH

———◆———

That is why athletes are important, why records are important. Because they demonstrate the scope of human possibility, which is unlimited. The inconceivable is conceived, and then it is accomplished.

— BRIAN GANVILLE, "THE OLYMPIAN"

———◆———

The starter had checked their identities now and was calling them to their positions . . . Colin felt his chest constrict and his mouth dry slightly; he was suddenly keyed-up. But not unpleasantly. He was the warhorse when it hears the bugle: there was going to be a fight and he was going to enjoy it. His skin began to prickle.

— VICTOR PRICE, "THE OTHER KINGDOM"

———◆———

When we understand the privilege of what it means to be an athlete, we are in touch with, and rejoice in, our physical, mental, and emotional strengths and our endless possibilities.

— GLORIA AVERBUCH

He felt good. Loose, with lots of juice in his flat-muscled body and an easy animal grace that brought the road back under him in long effortless strides.

— GEORGE HARMON COXE, "SEE HOW THEY RUN"

Although he was not a very good runner, he knew all about running.

— HARRY SYLVESTER, "GOING TO RUN ALL NIGHT"

Consistency requires discipline. Force yourself out the door.

— BOB GLOVER AND SHELLY-LYNN FLORENCE GLOVER, *THE COMPETITIVE RUNNER'S HANDBOOK*

When he hears the gun, his muscles will automatically spring to action. He can almost feel the breeze that will flow smoothly over his face and arms and legs. His spikes will rhythmically splash cinder behind him and there will be cheering from the bleachers to his right.

— LOUIS EDWARDS, "TEN SECONDS"

The feel of that day was still in his limbs: he remembered the vague glow of promise, the sense of being released as he sped over the turf of roughly prepared track—effortless, as though his body had lightened, brought to a pitch of harmony by the simple miracle of the up-drawing sun.

— GEORGE EWART EVANS, "THE MEDAL"

I don't consider hard work and great fun mutually exclusive. Who decided that anyway?

— DICK BEARDSLEY

———◆———

Experienced runners learn to respect the changing needs of their bodies. That's the wisdom that comes with time, and—for good or bad—with age.

— FRED LEBOW

———◆———

At first an ordeal and then an accomplishment, the daily run becomes a staple, like bread, or wine, a fine marriage, or air. It is also a free pass to friendship.

— BENJAMIN CHEEVER, *STRIDES*

———◆———

The runners would gather nervously at the starting line, taking care not to look each other in the eye.

— JOHN L. PARKER JR., *ONCE A RUNNER*

His body was a misery to him. He ran along beside the endless steel wire fence crying to himself, "Why did I think I could run! I can't! I'm not any good!"

— JAMES BUECHLER, "JOHN SOBIESKI BURNS"

[O]ne of the beautiful intangibles about runners is the bond we share. Like pregnant women, first-time dads, cancer patients, or recovering alcoholics, we share a deep-rooted commonality.

— GAIL W. KISLEVITZ

Out of a silver heat mirage he ran. Two lanes of blacktop stretched straight and flat in front of him, straight and flat behind. August-tall corn walled in the raod and its red-sand shoulders. A half mile away was a blue-dark wall of woods.

— JAMES TABOR, "THE RUNNER"

Running was the time he felt most alive. He knew that as surely as he'd ever known anything.

— RICHARD CHRISTIAN MATHESON, "THIRD WIND"

I waited for someone to speak, but all ran quietly, all alone. Now and then we would fall into step and there would be the thump thump thump of our running. Then the steps would syncopate and break rhythm and in the heavy depressing heat I would find myself having to concentrate to maintain stride.

— WALTER MCDONALD, "THE TRACK"

Maybe I'm a product of Wonder Woman comic books.

— NINA KUCSIK

———◆———

As yet there was no sensation of effort when he changed speed either up or down. He might have been advancing or retarding the starter handle of an electric motor.

— WILLIAM R. LOADER, "STAYING THE DISTANCE"

———◆———

I must have looked pretty scary, you know, when runners get that glazed look in their eyes, mouths covered in dried sweat, T-shirt soaked and ill-fitting.

— RICHARD BEL LICCHI

———◆———

His running had propriety, assurance; he possessed the event as, physically, his own.

— Douglas Dunn, "An Evening at the Track"

⸻

The town talk this day is of nothing but the great foot-race run this day on Banstead Downes, between Lee, the Duke of Richmond's footman, and Tyler, a famous runner. And Lee hath beaten him; though the King and Duke of York and all men almost did beat three or four to one upon the Tyler's head."

— Samuel Pepys's diary, July 30, 1663

⸻

I would give a thousand pound. I could run as fast as thou canst.

— Falstaff to Poins in Shakespeare's *Henry IV*

⸻

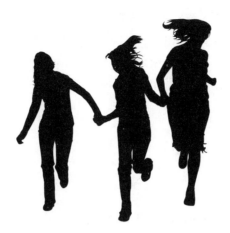

I couldn't admit this for many years, but I was afraid that if I took a break from running I'd lose it.

— DICK BEARDSLEY

————◆————

I ran all the way.

— HARRY S. TRUMAN, UPON RECEIVING A CALL ON APRIL 12, 1945 TO COME TO THE WHITE HOUSE

————◆————

We would start at the back of the meadow and run hell-bent to the ledge, stopping precariously close to our demise in order to embrace the wind hugging us back across our chests and under our outstretched arms. That was flying and I was immortal at that moment.

— KATE KINSEY

The only comfort I allowed myself was a run around the high school track. I'd go there in the after-school silence and run quietly, thinking of all the things I wanted to run away from. It was a moment of escape, a place where I could control everything—the distance I ran, how fast I would run, and where I was going.

— MARY HRICKO

I never responded to physical competition, internal or external, and preferred to run in the quiet of my own pace.

— SUZANNE CASE

When the gun shoots, you got to go.

> — ATO BOLDON

I ran to be free; I ran to avoid pain; I ran to feel pain; I ran out of love and hate and anger and joy.

> — DAGNY SCOTT, *RUNNERS WORLD COMPLETE BOOK OF WOMEN'S RUNNING*

I don't worry about what I've run. I worry about what I'm going to run. To be successful, you've got to keep moving.

> — RAE BAYMILLER

My outlook is that I never want to look back and wonder how fast I could have been.

> — DOUG MOCK

It's my own space, my own time, when I'm just out there letting my thoughts go. It's a part of my day like eating, and it's one of my favorite parts.

— LOUISE KENT

As a runner, you could compete and excel—you could calibrate just about every step that you took. Or you could throw away the damn watch, forget about competition, and use running to blow yourself out of your gourd.

— DAVID HOBLER

The main thing for me is to enjoy my running, just like it is for most people. Those long, slow runs—that's my time, my time to think.

— TRACEY HALLIDAY REUSCH

What makes running an integral part of someone's life? That may be an unanswerable question. Some people have no idea why they wake up every morning and have to get in their run.

— TOM FLEMING

I tell runners . . . that no matter how inexperienced a runner you may be, there is nothing wrong with being intense. You don't know what you might discover.

— FRANCIE LARRIEU SMITH

Running with your dog is probably one of the safest things you can do for yourself, and it can be great for the animal as well.

— MIMI NOONAN, DVM

In addition to the safety factor, we run together for companionship, and to remind each other how important a part of our lives this activity is.

— GORDON BLOCH

———⊰◆⊱———

Coaching is no different from what a choreographer does with a dance or what a playwright does with a play.

— BROOKS JOHNSON, STANFORD UNIVERSITY COACH

———⊰◆⊱———

My philosophy on running is, I don't dwell on it, I do it.

— JOAN SAMUELSON

———⊰◆⊱———

Everyone needs a good coach. That person is like an outside observer, another set of eyes.

— TOSHIKO D'ELIA

———⊰◆⊱———

As a coach, I try to keep people from taking their running too seriously.

— GORDON BLOCH

—◆—

I've been running for over 20 years; I read all the books and articles, yet I need a coach. Why? I still have to be told, to be encouraged.

— FRED LEBOW

—◆—

I have a few requirements about who I will coach. I think a person has to stay with a program at least one year. That's the only way to know if it works. If I sense an athlete won't stick with a program, I won't work with him or her.

— TOM FLEMING

—◆—

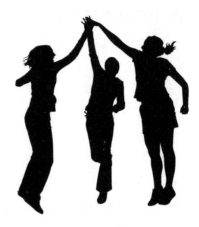

Most distance runners have good cardiovascular activity, but are lacking in overall athletic ability. Making a better athlete will automatically mean making a better runner.

— TRACY SUNDLUN, ASSISTANT COACH AT THE UNIVERSITY OF SOUTHERN CALIFORNIA

I definitely believe that an athlete is a good runner because he or she runs.

— TOM FLEMING

Free your mind, and your feet will follow.

— KEVIN NELSON, *THE RUNNER'S BOOK OF DAILY INSPIRATION*

My first year of running was spent going to road races around the New England area. I was welcomed by my fellow male runners, but often not by race promoters or race officials.

— CHARLOTTE LETTIS RICHARDSON

Our sport becomes not just what we do but an integral symbol—on all levels—of who we are.

— GLORIA AVERBUCH

The body loves variety. The body is the same as the seasons: It likes change.

— PRISCILLA WELCH

Everyone knows running is great for the cardiovascular system. However, it's also a fact that the sport dramatically tightens certain muscles while doing nothing for others.

— BERYL BENDER BIRCH

————◆————

Every athlete knows it's very hard to maintain consistency.

— BILL RODGERS

————◆————

Once I became sufficiently armed with the concept of overtraining, I began to do a little more research into this phenomenon. I soon uncovered that there were indeed some signs of doing too much, other than beginning a run and realizing your shorts were still in your dresser drawer. Nothing like standing in the middle of the road in your birthday suit to assist with the conclusion that you might be a tad overfatigued.

— BOB SCHWARTZ, *I RUN, THEREFORE I AM—NUTS*

————◆————

I'm conscious of every little pain and discomfort, from constipation to a side stitch. I have a new relationship to that pain. I don't fight it anymore; I respect my pain.

— FRED LEBOW

I have even cried once or twice when I crossed the finish line, out of a fullness of feeling that can't be expressed in words.

— LARRY SMITH

It's been proven that you can run, and run well, at age 40 and beyond. It's not merely a younger person's sport.

— PRISCILLA WELCH

Cross-country is my first great love in running. Like anyone's first love, I remember it with great sentimentality.

— LYNN JENNINGS

<hr/>

When the gun went off he sprang forward, running with long, ungainly strides which nevertheless ate up the ground in front of him. He finished yards ahead of the nearest runner. As he came back the crowd shouted with delight; but he paid little attention to them as he paced down the track with a slow dignity.

— GEORGE EWART EVANS, "THE MEDAL"

<hr/>

Sustained motivation is essential to achieving your potential.

— GRETE WAITZ

<hr/>

Success does not come to the most righteous and rigorously disciplined but to those who continue running.

— AMBY BURFOOT

———◆———

[I]t's only something normal for a sportsman to retire. You cannot control the whole world forever. People soon forget you because another champion comes along.

— HAILE GEBRSELASSIE

———◆———

I'm not doing what society dictates. I have no children. I run for a living.

— FRANCIE LARRIEU SMITH

———◆———

If it's fun and sweaty, just go out and do it.

— AMBY BURFOOT

———◆———

Sometimes, on days I'm truly not motivated, I use errands to make me run. I carry a plastic bag or small backpack and run to the store to shop.

— ANA DA SILVA

Running is my sunshine.

— JOAN TWINE

[O]n days when I'm not motivated, I reason that I'd rather put in one hour of drudgery to gain 23 hours of bliss. Bliss means that for the rest of the day, I'm not guilty about drinking a beer, watching a football game, taking a nap.

— STUART WITT

To really keep things light, at times I prefer silly running. I find a friend of similar temperament and we plan what I call bozo runs—like running with jingle bells on during Christmas season or costumes at Halloween.

— TOM ALLEN

———◆———

Bill Rodgers probably has more physical talent than anyone I've ever met, but his relaxed attitude under pressure is what distinguishes him.

— TOM FLEMING

———◆———

Some running should be different mentally just the way it is different physically. On my easy runs, I may use the time to relax and let my mind wander, but I never do that in hard workouts or races.

— GRETE WAITZ

———◆———

If you want to achieve a high goal, you're going to have to take some chances.

> — ALBERTO SALAZAR

What is the source of my success? I think it's a combination of consistency and balance.

> — MARK ALLEN

That day I learned that the race doesn't always go to the swift, but can go to the less fleet of foot (especially when they are the only ones running).

> — BOB SCHWARTZ, *I RUN, THEREFORE I AM—NUTS*

Sure I get nervous about competition. But I differentiate between being nervous and being uncontrollably nervous

— EAMONN COGHLAN

Prior to the 1991 New York City Marathon, I was walking down the street on the way to paint the blue line that runs along the course. I passed a pizza shop, and had a rare urge to indulge. It felt great. When it comes to food, I want to take advantage of every desire I have.

— FRED LEBOW

I've been asked if it's mental or physical ability that declines with age. I think it's mainly physical ability that changes, as opposed to any mental "burnout" that occurs from being at it for years.

— BILL RODGERS

I think it's an ego trip. I'm a show-off. If I had done all this at age 50, no one would have paid any attention.

— LOIS SCHEFFELIN, 80-YEAR-OLD MARATHON RUNNER

If people are physically fit, they are better adjusted for life.

— AL GORDON, 90-YEAR-OLD ATHLETE

Running has enormous psychological and physical benefits, especially for women in the older age categories. It celebrates your age and your ability.

— ANNA THORNHILL, 52-YEAR-OLD ARTIST

I am very involved with my grandchildren now, which means so much to my pleasure. I am happy to adjust my training regime to spend time with them. This has helped me to accept my aging as it relates to my running.

— TOSHIKA D'ELIA, 62-YEAR-OLD MARATHONER

I started blooming when I was 40.

— PRISCILLA WELCH

———◆———

Through running I experience my own epiphany, a manifestation of the essential nature of who I am, the man I want to be.

— MATTHEW SHAFNER

———◆———

There is untold fulfillment to be gained from the sport.

— NINA KUSCSIK

———◆———

I hope my children remember me being in my prime as a mother, not as a runner.

— JOAN SAMUELSON

———◆———

Movement is almost synonymous with life.

— BERND HEINRICH, *WHY WE RUN: A NATURAL HISTORY*

———◆———

When you run in places you visit, you encounter things you'd never see otherwise.

— TOM BROKAW

———◆———

At eighteen miles the lead runners began to catch up with me, whizzing by as if I was going backward. Bill Rodgers passed me by, yelling, "Thataboy, Dick." That had to be one of the most exciting thrills of my life.

— DICK TRAUM, THE FIRST AMPUTEE TO RUN THE NEW YORK CITY MARATHON

———◆———

There were no spectators, only goats. I actually have a special feeling for goats, as we used to have them at home when I was growing up. But they don't make for a great cheering section.

— FRED LEBOW ON RUNNING THE ARUBA MARATHON

I loved cross country right from the start. I loved the open territory and going the distance.

— BILL RODGERS

You're . . . better off having the same attitude in business as you have for successful running.

— ALBERTO SALAZAR

The days of running in good old-fashioned sweats—as in sweatshirts and sweatpants—are woefully numbered, and for good reason.

— DON MOGELEFSKY

⸻

If you can take the banging and jostling, running is one of the best possible ways to work out for skinniness.

— *THE SKINNY: WHAT EVERY SKINNY WOMAN KNOWS ABOUT DIETING (AND WON'T TELL YOU!)*, PATRICIA MARX AND SUSAN SISTROM

⸻

Thrust against pain. Pain is the purifier.

— PERCY CERUTTY

⸻

Many women take up running to lose weight—with good reason, since running is one of the most efficient and best calorie-burning activities around. What often happens, though, is that once a woman begins running, she discovers many rewards she didn't expect.

— CLAIRE KOWALCHIK, *THE COMPLETE BOOK OF RUNNING FOR WOMEN*

I can only run a 10-minute mile, but I don't care about that. I like to run first thing in the morning because it makes me feel really good and gives me more energy for the rest of the day.

— KATHY DOUKAS

I waited a long time to start running because I didn't think I could run fast enough. When I started running at "only" four-and-a-half miles per hour, a whole new world opened up.

— ALLISON PROCTOR

Your first goal is to avoid getting trampled by the crowd.

— BOB GLOVER AND SHELLY-LYNN FLORENCE GLOVER, *THE
COMPETITIVE RUNNER'S HANDBOOK*

———◆———

I love the Olympics. . . . If this was any other race, I would pull out. But
the Ethiopian people expect me to run. . . . I have to think about that, too.
Athens is not only for myself.

— HAILE GEBRSELASSIE ON THE 2004 SUMMER OLYMPICS IN ATHENS

———◆———

The mind is always selling the body.

— JOHN LANDY

———◆———

He was going to grind the opposition into the earth, and if he ground himself in the process, that was too bad.

— WILLIAM R. LOADER, "STAYING THE DISTANCE"

Running prowess may seem unimportant to an antelope until that rare moment in its life when a lion gives chase.

— BERND HEINRICH, *WHY WE RUN: A NATURAL HISTORY*

Walking or running makes us part of the living cosmic unity, and that is not something restricted to the young.

— ROGER ROBINSON

No man would deny that a thoroughly healthy state of body is the normal and most essential condition of athletic excellence. And just the same thing may be said of spiritual and intellectual health.

— CHARLES KINGSLEY

We are constantly astonished by mature runners who defy the dictates of age. Their secret? It often seems to be a youthful spirit and an active mind.

— RHONDA PROVOST

Commitment to the body machine. It was as critical as the commitment to the goal itself.

— RICHARD CHRISTIAN MATHESON, "THIRD WIND"

One of my biggest desires as a coach is to help adults learn to run like they did as kids. It's such a natural movement when kids do it.

— T'AI CHI MASTER GEORGE XU

In Antarctica you don't just need physical strength. You also need courage and wisdom.

— WILLIAM TAN, WHEELCHAIR PARTICIPANT IN THE ANTARCTICA MARATHON

You can jog while pushing a baby carriage.

— NINA KUCSIK

The numbers are in and they show women's running is hot.

— GLORIA AVERBUCH

Years ago, women sat in kitchens drinking coffee and discussing life. Today, they cover the same topics while they run.

— JOAN BENOIT SAMUELSON

The way I see it, you have to view running time not as extra or wasted time, but as important, productive contemplation time.

— FRED LEBOW

Gazelles run when they're pregnant. Why should it be any different for women?

— JOAN ULLYOT, M.D.

The best parent of a young runner is supportive and approving, but leaves the logistics of training and racing to others.

— JOHN BABINGTON, LIBERTY ATHLETIC CLUB COACH AND ASSISTANT COACH FOR THE 1996 OLYMPIC WOMEN'S TRACK-AND-FIELD TEAM

———◆———

There are other reasons, besides training, why things change; life intervenes.

— FRANCIE LARRIEU SMITH

———◆———

Knowing that you can run 20 miles is a big breakthrough mentally, when it comes to tackling the marathon distance.

— JOAN BENOIT SAMUELSON

———◆———

Don't automatically head for a high-tech shoe. I think you should only wear as much shoe as you need for your body to work as efficiently as it can.

— TOM HARTGE, NIKE

Use goals not as ends in themselves but as stepping stones. When you reach 80 percent of your long-range goal, reset it.

— DR. LINDA BUNKER, SPORTS PSYCHOLOGIST

Success is 90 percent physical and 10 percent mental. But never underestimate the power of that 10 percent.

— TOM FLEMING

Classical antiquity knew no such race as the marathon.

— Andrew Suozzo, *The Chicago Marathon*

———◆———

My only concern was to go as fast as I could and I was rewarded with my best personal marathon record.

— Rosa Mota on the 1984 Chicago Marathon

———◆———

I looked up at the time with the seconds ticking off and, with the wind blowing in my face, I gave it one final burst because I felt the record was in my grasp.

— Steve Jones on the 1984 Chicago Marathon

———◆———

You don't want your competition to know what's ailing you.

— DICK BEARDSLEY

———◆———

Ultimately, the best runners are the ones who are willing to work very hard but who have a little bit of a lazy streak in them.

— BENJI DURDEN, COACH

———◆———

Somewhere along the path, running became the canvas upon which I documented my life.

— DAGNY SCOTT, *RUNNERS WORLD COMPLETE BOOK OF WOMEN'S RUNNING*

———◆———

I race in order to dig deep within myself and see what I'm really made of.

— MAGGIE, RUNNER FROM IDAHO

We must wake up to the fact that athletics is not, nor ever can be perfected; there will always be more to learn.

— ARTHUR "GREATHEART" NEWTON, 1949

For me and many others, it is simply more than we could stand.

— CHRIS CHATAWAY ON TRAINING REGIMES OF EMIL ZATOPEK AND JOHN LANDY

I don't think anyone can be so self-sufficient that they don't feel the need for somebody else.

— CHRIS BRASHER ON THE IMPORTANCE OF A COACH

We've suffered the pain, felt the glory, and, when all the sweat is spent, we have the faith to reach deep inside to find that ounce of energy left in our heels, our heart, our soul, to carry us across the finish line stiff-legged and fatigue-racked, but with a smile of victory.

— GAIL W. KISLEVITZ

The ability to make a man go beyond the point at which he thinks he is going to die.

— FRANZ STAMPFL ON WHAT COACHES NEED

I felt at that moment that it was my chance to do one thing supremely well.

— ROGER BANNISTER

———◆———

When you run in the morning, you gain time in a sense. It's like stretching 24 hours into 25. You may need to sleep less and get up earlier, but if you can get by that, running early seems to expand the day.

— FRED LEBOW

———◆———

There's nothing a man can't do if the spirit's there.

— FRANZ STAMPFL

———◆———

The surprising part is that women are usually more sensible than men. I find this in their approach to sports in general . . . they seem more willing to listen to so-called voices of authority, or reason.

— GORDON BLOCH

Running is not only physical. If it were, you could put a great bull-like guy to it and he'd break every record.

— DENIS JOHANSSON

Given the nature of running, certain things will never be altered. That's one of the beauties of our sport. There is no judge; it doesn't matter how you look.

— BILL RODGERS

I love the feeling of cross country running, because it's done in the elements. The footing is tough and you're running against nature.

— Lynn Jennings

⬥

Jogging on the shores of the Black Sea in Varna in Bulgaria, I passed another runner. I didn't speak his language. He didn't speak mine. "Paavo Nurmi," I called out. "Paavo Nurmi," he called back.

— Benjamin Cheever, *Strides*

⬥

Those who are self-coached can become stagnant or bored. At least occasionally, it might be good for those people to seek out some coaching advice.

— Francie Larrieu Smith

⬥

When I started running after the birth of my daughter, I had over 50 pounds to lose. What helped me greatly was constant positive reinforcement. I didn't think of myself as a fat runner because I knew that such negative thinking wasn't going to help me to lose the weight.

— Florence Griffith Joyner

All I want to do is speed, speed.

— Miki Gorman

We train and compete year round, and running is worldwide. Running is very different from other sports in that regard.

— Bill Rodgers

Something in me wanted to find out how far I could run without stopping.

— JACKI HANSON

⸻⬦⸻

The astonishing white soles of his feet rise and salute us on the turns.

— MAXINE W. KUMIN

⸻⬦⸻

I think I've been good, but I want to be better. I think women reach their peak in their mid-thirties.

— MARY DECKER SLANEY

⸻⬦⸻

The only way I was going to make a difference for myself or any other black person is to say the hurdles were there and do what I had to do.

— WYOMIA TYUS

I don't stop until the world gets gray and fuzzy around the edges.

— CANDI CLARK

Do they tackle you in cross-country?

— DICK BEARDSLEY TO A FRIEND IN HIGH SCHOOL

Accept your limitation and, with care, the thinking runner will have a comfortable, creditable race. But go for broke and prepare to be broken.

— GEORGE SHEEHAN

It turned out that no one without the standard issue of two working legs had ever run a marathon before. It took me seven hours and twenty-four minutes to finish and the excitement generated at that race hasn't stopped yet.

— DICK TRAUM ON RUNNING THE NEW YORK CITY MARATHON IN 1976

The history of women's competitive racing can be traced back to ancient Greece, when every five years a short footrace was held at a women's festival to honor the Greek goddess Hera.

— SHANTI SOSIENSKI, *WOMEN WHO RUN*

Running was a practical and mystical discipline. It was a way of melding the inner and outer realms.

— DAVID HOBLER

You feel good while you're running and you feel even better when you're finished.

— FRED LEBOW

I taught my guys to constantly change their move patterns. For instance, the natural tendency of a runner is to rest once he climbs to the top of a hill. My athletes would get to the top of a hill, fake like they were going to lay down and die, and then take off. It would catch the other guy with his thumb up his butt.

— BILL SQUIRES

Running has filled many unforgiving minutes for me.

— MATTHEW SHAFNER

Did the cat do stretches? Did the cat jog around? Did the cat do knee bends? Did the cat have a track suit on before racing? No, the cat just got up and went. No more warming up. Forget it.

— PERCY CERUTTY TO HIS TEAM AFTER DUMPING A BUCKET OF WATER ON A CAT AND WATCHING IT RUN AWAY

Squires said the more you can get your body used to accelerating, then backing off, then flying up and down hills, then recovering, then sprinting—the more you do this kind of thing in practice, the more ready you are when you get in a race.

— DICK BEARDSLEY ON BILL SQUIRES

[Running] transported him, taking his mind to another place, very deep within. Like prayer.

— RICHARD CHRISTIAN MATHESON, "THIRD WIND"

A lot of people asked me, "Well, are you going to be scared to push yourself again?" I wasn't. That fall, I broke through tremendously.

— ALBERTO SALAZAR ON THE 1978 FALMOUTH RACE WHERE HE BECAME
SO DEHYDRATED THAT HE WAS ADMINISTERED LAST RITES

There are . . . some horrifying warnings being issued that [running] might break down the collagen in your face (all that bouncing, we guess) which would result in a very saggy profile, but we'll keep running until that's a proven fact and anyway, isn't that what facelifts are for?

— *THE SKINNY: WHAT EVERY SKINNY WOMAN KNOWS ABOUT DIETING (AND WON'T TELL YOU!)*, PATRICIA MARX AND SUSAN SISTROM

He ticked off six miles with reaching strides, his rhythm rolling on itself, like coasting downhill on oiled bearings.

— JAMES TABOR, "THE RUNNER"

Many manufacturers are competing for your foot.

— SYBIL ROBINSON

A journey of a thousand miles begins with a single step.

— CHINESE PROVERB

The beginning is the chiefest part of any work.

— PLATO

—❖—

For years, I've been in the habit of wearing running shoes everywhere and for every function. I even wear them with my tuxedo.

— FRED LEBOW

—❖—

I don't—and, on most days, don't believe I even can—sweat without my earbuds firmly in place.

— DIMITY MCDOWELL

—❖—

Compared to a lot of runners, I'm not very loyal to my running shoes.

— SARAH BOWEN SHEA

———◈———

Running has always helped keep me sane, so I thought running could help these guys burn off energy and stress.

— LAURA BOWMAN, WHO IS IN CHARGE OF A RUNNING CLUB FOR
PRISONERS

———◈———

He lived only for running. He got up in the morning and walked to the school for it, waiting all day for that living half hour when he emerged on the playing field and ran, suffering, until he swore he would never do it again, and at last finished somehow and returned to the locker room.

— JAMES BUECHLER, "JOHN SOBIESKI BURNS"

———◈———

Running has given me an opportunity to reach out and be a benefit to a fellow human being.

— MARK GOLDSTEIN ON THE KOMEN RACE FOR THE CURE, A 5K THAT RAISES BREAST CANCER AWARENESS

Most runners want to run either longer or faster at some point in their running career, but without good running form, added distance will only lengthen the time you are running improperly and increase your odds of getting hurt.

— GEORGE XU

I'm just doing what I love to do—swimming, biking, running—whether I have legs or not. If I had legs, I might not be as active.

— RUDY GARCIA-TOLSON, WHO CAN RUN A 5.57-MINUTE MILE ON TWO PROSTHETIC LEGS

Running is the space in my day when I feel the most beautiful—when I don't feel judged by others. And that's what I want for all little girls.

— MOLLY BARKER, FOUNDER OF GIRLS ON THE RUN INTERNATIONAL

My eyes burned with sweat, and I squinted so tight I could hardly see anymore, and because they stung it was impossible to think. I was adjusting, though, lost in rhythm, like a mechanical animal caught on the rim of existence . . . it felt good and I was slipping deep in dreams.

— WALTER MCDONALD, "THE TRACK"

I give my staff my running schedule six months in advance. God help them if they put something on top of it.

— FORMER ARKANSAS GOVERNOR MIKE HUCKABEE

I tried to use what notoriety and credibility I built for good things.

— FRANK SHORTER

◆

Before Prozac, the fastest pace I could run was about 5:20 per mile, and even doing that killed me. Three days after I began taking Prozac, I ran a workout of three 1-mile repeats. I did each of them in 5 minutes, comfortably. A few days later, I did a 6-by-1 mile workout at 4:42 per mile.

— ALBERTO SALAZAR

◆

When you have the enthusiasm and the passion, you end up figuring how to excel.

— DEENA KASTOR

◆

How much happiness is gained, and how much misery escaped, by frequent and violent agitation of the body.

— SAMUEL JOHNSON

I think there is a correlation between running and business success.

— ALBERTO SALAZAR

It is the illusion that we can go no faster that holds us back.

— KENNY MOORE

Running is a gift I give myself almost every day. Even on those days when things haven't gone great, I can come home and give myself the accomplishment of a 30- or 40-minute run.

—ARTHUR BLANK

Spend at least some of your training time, and other parts of your day, concentrating on what you are doing in training and visualizing your success.

— GRETE WAITZ

Run into peace.

— MEISTER ECKHART, 14TH-CENTURY PHILOSOPHER

When you run, you log on to yourself. You flip through the pages of your being.

— KEVIN NELSON, *THE RUNNER'S BOOK OF DAILY INSPIRATION*

When it's pouring rain and you're bowling along through the wet, there's satisfaction in knowing you're out there and the others aren't.

— PETER SNELL

To get to the finish line, you'll have to try lots of different paths.

— AMBY BURFOOT

Keep varying the program. Your body will tell you what to do.

— JOAN BENOIT

Play not only keeps us young but also maintains our perspective about the relative seriousness of things. Running is play, for even if we try hard to do well at it, it is a relief from everyday cares.

— JIM FIXX

Always stretch your hamstrings before you run. Spend a half hour on it. Stretch those hamstrings especially.

— DEANDRA CARTER

Running should be a lifelong activity. Approach it patiently and intelligently, and it will reward you for a long, long time.

— MICHAEL SARGENT

The conclusion I've come to after teaching countless runners is that *running does not hurt your body*.

— GEORGE XU

I'm willing to accept any kind of pain to win a race.

— RICK WOHLHUTTER

Running gives me confidence.

— STEVE PREFONTAINE

As athletes—even just by who we are and how we live—we are able to pass on a great gift to other women and girls.

— GLORIA AVERBUCH

I felt like I could see and hear everything. When I crossed the finish line that afternoon, I felt glorious, like I was going to live forever.

— DAVID HOBLER ON THE 1982 BOSTON MARATHON

My body immediately reacts to a lack of exercise. "Take me outside," it cries, "let me out."

— PAULA ZAHN

———◆———

I was hurting from sheer physical exhaustion, but when I heard the cheering, it carried me along. I wasn't going to stop now. The last quarter mile, when the crowds were at their peak, they roared as if I was running down a football field for the winning touchdown.

— DICK TRAUM, THE FIRST AMPUTEE TO RUN THE NEW YORK CITY MARATHON

———◆———

So much in life seems inflexible and unchangeable, and part of the joy of running and especially racing is the realization that improvement and progress can be achieved.

— NANCY ANDERSON

———◆———

I love running because you feel so good.

— BARBARA ORR

I knew I had disciplined myself, that running was my own doing. I knew that no one had pushed me to do it. I knew that I was able to accomplish what I had because I had worked on it.

— NINA KUSCIK

Life is complicated. Running is simple. Is it any wonder that people like to run?

— KEVIN NELSON, *THE RUNNER'S BOOK OF DAILY INSPIRATION*

If you become restless, speed up. If you become winded, slow down. You climb the mountain in a equilibrium between restlessness and exhaustion.

— ROBERT PIRSIG

I have two doctors: my left leg and my right.

— GEORGE M. TREVELYAN

It is better, I think, to begin easily and get your running to be smooth and relaxed and then to go faster and faster.

— HENRY RONO

Methinks that the moment my legs began to move, my thoughts began to flow.

— HENRY DAVID THOREAU

Cross country is like being a mountain goat, picking your way over roots and rocks, leaping over logs. It's grueling; it takes a lot of heart. But the rewards are great.

— LYNN JENNINGS

Mountains should be climbed with as little effort as possible and without desire. The reality of your own nature should determine the speed.

— ROBERT PIRSIG

Many people shy away from hills. They make it easy on themselves, but that limits their improvement. The more you repeat something, the stronger you get.

— JOE CATALANO

After a week of the contained chaos that is my job, I need some solitary running time. On Sundays, I can unwind and reconnect with the natural world.

— LINDA JONES

———◆———

It's best to approach your break point without breaking it.

— LEE FIDLER, RUNNING COACH

———◆———

Running long and hard is an ideal antidepressant, since it's hard to run and feel sorry for yourself at the same time. Also, there are those hours of clearheadedness that follow a long run.

— MONTE DAVIS

———◆———

We are what we repeatedly do. Excellence, then, is not an act, but a habit.

— ARISTOTLE

———◆———

There's nothing quite like the feeling you get from knowing you're in good physical condition. I wake up alert and singing in the morning, ready to go.

— STAN GERSTEIN

———◆———

The sanity of runners is also called into question, since we can sometimes be found slowly moving up and down the driveway while staring at a watch.

— BOB SCHWARTZ, *I RUN, THEREFORE I AM—NUTS*

———◆———

There are days for the paved streets and the track, days when you must follow the normal course traveled by other runners. Then there are days when you leave the beaten path behind you and run cross-country across the top of a ridge.

— KEVIN NELSON, *THE RUNNER'S BOOK OF DAILY INSPIRATION*

———◆———

[W]hether or not the International Olympic Committee has recognized it, women have always found a way to run.

— SHANTI SOSIENSKI, *WOMEN WHO RUN*

———◆———

I was hardly able to know that my legs were lifting and falling and my arms going in and out, and my lungs didn't seem to be working at all, and my heart stopped that wicked thumping I always get at the beginning of a run.

— ALAN SILLITOE, "THE LONELINESS OF THE LONG-DISTANCE RUNNER"

———◆———

I had always been active. When I was growing up, if I saw a green grassy field, I had this upwelling of joy. I would run across it with my arms up in the air. I couldn't help myself. It was a love of life.

— BOBBI GIBB

In 1970 when I started running there were very few opportunities for women runners to compete at longer distances. We could run the 880 and the mile, but not much further.

— CHARLOTTE LETTIS RICHARDSON

The first time I heard the word "marathon" I was a sophomore in high school and saw a picture of Ellison "Tarzan" Brown, who had won the 1936 and 1939 Boston Marathons. He was a dark-skinned Indian and at first, I thought he was another black runner.

— TED CORBITT

I knew that women were capable of running marathons if they were only given the opportunity.

— KATHRINE SWITZER

⎯⎯◆⎯⎯

The runner's greatest asset, apart from essential fitness of body, is a cool and calculating brain allied to confidence and courage.

— FRANZ STAMPFL, *FRANZ STAMPFL ON RUNNING*

⎯⎯◆⎯⎯

Get out of my race!

— BOSTON MARATHON OFFICIAL JOCK SEMPLE TO KATHRINE SWITZER IN 1967

⎯⎯◆⎯⎯

Passion is running and running is passion.

— GAIL W. KISLEVITZ

⎯⎯◆⎯⎯

The confident Hare took off at top speed . . . lollopped along, feeling pleased with its own brilliance . . . and stopped for a nap. . . . The determined Tortoise kept patiently padding and plodding along without any pause, until quietly it waddled past the sleeping Hare.

— AESOP

We don't let any grass grow under our feet, we're too busy running!

— KIM AHRENS

I knew if I quit, nobody would ever believe that women had the capability to run the marathon distance.

— KATHRINE SWITZER

The man who is in the state of running, of continuous running into peace, is a heavenly man. He continually runs and moves and seeks peace in running.

— MEISTER ECKHART

I hope to be the fastest fat old git in the race.

— EAMONN MARTIN, BEFORE WINNING THE 1993 LONDON MARATHON

Not unless they have Dutch elm disease.

— ROBDE CASTELLA, ON BEING ASKED WHETHER HAVING "TREE TRUNKS FOR LEGS" WAS A DISADVANTAGE IN RUNNING MARATHONS

Scratch marathoners once, they tell you how wonderful they feel. Scratch them twice and they tell you about their latest injuries.

— ARNOLD COOPER

You don't run 26 miles at five miles a minute on good looks and a secret recipe.

— FRANK SHORTER

I am still looking for shoes that will make running on streets seem like running barefoot across the bosoms of maidens.

— DAVE BROSNAN

That day remains very special to me and if I had one day to live over in my lifetime, it would be my first marathon.

— DICK TRAUM, THE FIRST AMPUTEE TO RUN THE NEW YORK CITY MARATHON

I have always sensed the exhilaration and independence of being self-propelled.

— NINA KUCSIK

⟫⟶⟫⟶⟫

The day I walk into the home of any runner in any African city, town, or village and find a StairMaster, rowing machine, or wet vest near a swimming pool, I'll be proved wrong. Until that day, I stick by my belief in the need to concentrate on putting in the running miles.

— TOM FLEMING

⟫⟶⟫⟶⟫

There is no path I follow. I feel as if I'm just drifting along, because although I can progress physically, through my training, mentally and spiritually I don't know what the hell I'm doing. It's like that car sticker: "Don't follow me, I'm lost."

— STEVE OVETT

The French cannot produce great track-and-field teams like they can produce great wines for probably that reason: the winemakers got in first.

— MICHAEL LOURIE

———◆———

Haile is a man with a social conscience. . . . He is arguably one of the greatest athletes of all time and, like Muhammad Ali, his impact on society and individuals transcends sport.

— GARETH DAVIS ON HAILE GEBRSELASSIE, IN THE *DAILY TELEGRAPH*

———◆———

When I run, my mind and body fuse together, creating an energy source that empowers me.

— GAIL W. KISLEVITZ

———◆———

The I'm-going-to-win-no-matter-how-I-have-to-do-it attitude just doesn't seem to fit. For me, a contest isn't a success unless it was fun, whether or not I win.

— Margo Godfrey Oberg

———◆———

The more energy you expend in running, the more energy you have.

— Kevin Nelson, *The Runner's Book of Daily Inspiration*

———◆———

I knew I had to do it. It was an order from the coach.

— Charlotte Smith

———◆———

Scientific testing on the benefits of vitamin, mineral, and herbal preparations is inconclusive at best. This lack of absolute proof doesn't turn runners away from these products. They work because we use the strongest additive of all—faith.

— JOE HENDERSON, *RUNNING 101*

For every runner who tours the world running marathons, there are thousands who run to hear the leaves and listen to the rain, and look to the day when it is suddenly as easy as a bird in flight.

— GEORGE SHEEHAN

I've been running a lot of open races against Kenyans and they like to blow it out hard in the beginning . . . it's a little scary doing that because you can just die out there doing that.

— MIKE MYKYTOK

When I run with someone else, the conversation flows naturally because
. . . what else can we do?

— AMBY BURFOOT, *THE RUNNER'S GUIDE TO THE MEANING OF LIFE*

Almost thirty years ago, I lined up for my first marathon. Little did I
know then how much that event would change my life.

— GRETE WAITZ, *RUN YOUR FIRST MARATHON*

No, Jackie, this isn't a coach-athlete thing. This is your husband telling
you its time for you to go

— BOB KERSEE, COACH TO JACKIE JOYNER-KERSEE, ASKING HER TO
RETIRE

If you train intelligently and have the right gear, you can continue to enjoy the fitness and general sense of well-being that accompanies running while avoiding running injuries.

— *THE U.S. NAVY SEAL GUIDE TO FITNESS AND NUTRITION*

———◆———

These frenzied spectators literally overwhelmed him, swarming round, shouting, yelling, dancing and jumping about like madmen. Those who got near him slapped and banged him on the back, yelling as they did so, "Good!" "Splendid!" "Glorious!" Thus they continued until all the little remaining breath in George's body was well-nigh beaten out of him.

— ACCOUNT FROM AN UNNAMED NEWSPAPER ABOUT WALTER GOODALL GEORGE'S VICTORY IN A RUNNING EVENT WITH WILLIAM CUMMINGS IN ENGLAND IN 1886.

———◆———

Pain is a given. I don't try to fight the pain or pretend it's not there. In fact, I give into it. But only for a little while.

— RIC MUNOZ

The marathon has been referred to as a person's horizontal Everest.

— GRETE WAITZ AND GLORIA AVERBUCH, *RUN YOUR FIRST MARATHON*

———◆———

I'm rapidly getting to the point now where I don't care about the interviews or anything anymore. I guess from a business point of view every bit of publicity you can get is good, but it's just not worth it to me. You get sick about talking about the same thing over and over again.

— ALBERTO SALAZAR

———◆———

It was a lifetime of training for just 10 seconds.

— JESSE OWENS, ON THE OLYMPICS

———◆———

Don't let anybody kid you. Runners make runners. Coaches like to take all the credit, but day after day, the upper classmen show the younger fellows how to run, how to train, how to take care of themselves.

— JUMBO ELLIOT

———◆◆◆———

Winning is always satisfying, but when you succeed in a marathon, it stays with you. . .You will feel the sweetness of the achievement forever.

— GRETE WAITZ AND GLORIA AVERBUCH, *RUN YOUR FIRST MARATHON*

———◆◆◆———

Everyone knows about the bear. He's that invisible animal that waits for you about a hundred yards from the finish line. He jumps on your back and starts clawing and scratching and he seems so heavy that you want to stop running so that he'll get off and leave you alone.

— BRUCE JENNER

———◆◆◆———

CHAPTER FOURTEEN

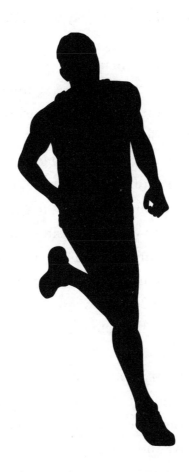

On the marathon and beyond

Going the Distance

With a half dozen miles to go in a marathon, Frank Shorter commented to friendly rival Kenny Moore, "Too bad Pheidippides didn't die at 20 miles."

But would the magic of the marathon remain if the distance had been anything less than the admittedly quirky 26 miles 385 yards? Would we still see nearly 40,000 runners lined up on starting lines from Chicago to New York to London to Berlin?

Possibly, but if we appeased Frank and lowered the bar, it would remove from the race a significant challenge. Scientists tell us that we can store enough glycogen in our muscles to get us to the 20-mile mark, the so-called "Wall." Those who train using one of my programs get to that distance in their last long run and stop without significantly having tested themselves. Intermediate and Advanced runners following my programs run two or three 20-milers. More experienced marathoners run somewhat more often than that, elite runners going that far week after week after week.

But move into that 21st mile, and the 22nd, and the 23rd, and the ones beyond, and it is like punching the button on the treadmill that elevates the belt. Parts start coming off the machine: your machine!

Yes, Frank. Let's leave the distance alone. In your victory at the Olympic Games in Munich, there remained still a few speedy runners in your wake who might have stayed with you had the distance been a more mortal 20 miles. By 26 miles 385 yards, there remained no doubt who was champion that day.

And as runners today cross the finish line at that magical distance, they continue to join you on the victory stand.

If you want to win something, run 100 meters. If you want to experience something, run a marathon.

— EMIL ZATOPEK

———◆———

When I run a marathon, I put myself at the center of my life, the center of my universe. For these hours, I move past ideas of food and shelter and sexual fulfillment and other basic drives.

— GEORGE SHEEHAN

———◆———

He was thinking: There is nothing like the Marathon. Just the figures alone mean something: 26 miles, 385 yards.

— JOHN L. PARKER, JR., *ONCE A RUNNER*

———◆———

Aretha Franklin's "Respect" started playing. In my head, I was singing, "R-E-S-P-E-C-T" and suddenly I got that last nudge through the finish.

> — JOHN-LOUIS KRONFELD, ON BREAKING THROUGH "THE WALL" AT THE MARINE CORPS MARATHON

Your goal is to keep an even pace or, even better, to speed up at the end, running so-called negative splits. Most runners do the opposite, with devastating results. Every recent world best in the marathon was set by athletes who ran at an even pace or ran negative splits.

> — GINA KOLATA, "KEEPING THE GAUGE OFF 'E,'" *THE NEW YORK TIMES,* OCTOBER 25, 2007

Years ago, the picture of people running marathons was these lean, mean Type-A male running machines, but today people running are your neighbors, just regular people. It's a different sport now and we have to cater to these new people, not exclude them.

> — TRACY SUNDLUN, EXECUTIVE VICE PRESIDENT OF ELITE RACING, ON OPPOSING THE BAN ON USING HEADPHONES IN RACES

Runners are no longer content with fitness but are seeking a new awareness of the self in the total experience of running—and more often than not they are culminating that quest by running a marathon.

— GEORGE SHEEHAN

Every serious marathoner should do Boston, to experience the close to a million spectators, the three generations of families out cheering, the little kids handing you water or orange slices. The whole city really appreciates the runners.

— NEIL WEYGANDT, WHO HAD FINISHED 41 STRAIGHT BOSTON MARATHONS AS OF 2007

The marathon had always been a hand-me-down kind of event. In general, guys went into the marathon because they weren't fast enough at the shorter distances.

— BILL SQUIRES ON MARATHONS IN THE 1970s

If people were possessed by reason, running marathons would not work. But we are not creatures of reason. We are creatures of passion.

— NOEL CARROLL

I used to be a runner myself, quite a useful one too but a bit of a plodder.

— ALLAN SILLITOE, *THE LONELINESS OF THE LONG DISTANCE RUNNER*

Carbo-loading will only get you twenty miles. For the last six you eat your heart out. In my training, even with Gatorade and bee pollen and seventy-dollar heel inserts, I can't make it past twenty miles.

— MAX APPLE, "CARBO-LOADING"

A miler's kick does the trick. . . . A miler's kick does the trick. . .

> — Rod Dixon's mental refrain as he chased down and beat
> Geoff Smith in the last half mile of the 1983 New York City
> Marathon

No doubt a brain and some shoes are essential for marathon success, although if it comes down to a choice, pick the shoes. More people finish marathons with no brains than with no shoes.

> — Don Kardong

Never stand directly in front of a runner after they've finished a marathon. It's a mistake you make only once—and it'll cost you a pair of shoes.

> — John Bingham, "You're in Good Hands," *Runners World*

It is important to keep the marathon in perspective. Running does not have to be the controlling element in your life, but if you become a marathon runner it probably will be, for a while.

— MARC BLOOM, *THE RUNNER'S BIBLE*

—❦—

The marathon . . . is, to use Yeats's description of poetry, "blood, imagination, and intellect brought together."

— GEORGE SHEEHAN

—❦—

[I]n an unequal world, in this one endeavor people of vastly differing abilities share something in common: the act of going the distance. Whether it's two hours or four or five, the effort and achievement are similar.

— FRED LEBOW

—❦—

The distance race is a struggle that results in self-discovery. It is an adventure involving the limits of the self.

— PAUL WEISS

The difference between the mile and the marathon is the difference between burning your fingers with a match and being slowly roasted over hot coals.

— HAL HIGDON, "ON THE RUN FROM DOGS AND PEOPLE"

Runners have died in marathons all over the world, most commonly from heart ailments, dehydration and over-hydration. [Dr. Lewis Maharam, the medical director of the New York Marathon] said statistics showed a death happens once every 50,000 to 75,000 competitors.

— LYNN ZINSER & MICHAEL S. SCHMIDT, "READY TO RACE, REMINDED OF RISKS," *THE NEW YORK TIMES,* NOVEMBER 4, 2007

What is the great appeal of the marathon? This is something I continually ask myself as nearly 50,000 requests for entries pour in every year for the New York City Marathon.

— FRED LEBOW

Running a marathon is a tremendous accomplishment. I never understood why people ran them until I did it. Crossing the finish line of my first marathon gave me that "first-time glow"—a sense of accomplishment that I have not felt since.

— FRANCIE LARRIEU SMITH

The marathon is a bizarre event, and as a coach I hate it.

— BOB SEVENE

At no other course did I stand on the start and feel my arms tingle.

— GREG MEYER ON THE BOSTON MARATHON, WHICH HE WON IN 1983

I thought about how many preconceived prejudices would crumble when I trotted right along for 26 miles.

— ROBERTA "BOBBI" GIBB

Is that where women go in childbirth—into the place of charms? All gay women should run marathons—gives them solidarity with their laboring sisters.

— SARA MAITLAND, "THE LOVELINESS OF THE LONG-DISTANCE RUNNER"

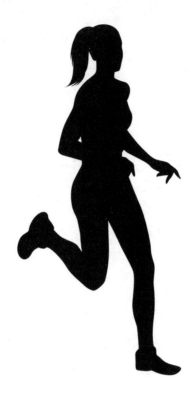

I don't train to beat another runner. We are out there together, competing with the marathon, and I train to run the marathon as fast as I can.

— JUMA IKANGAA

Almost every first-time marathoner says the same thing at the finish line: "Never again."

— BOB GLOVER, *THE RUNNER'S HANDBOOK*

I viewed every marathon as a test of my manhood.

— ALBERTO SALAZAR

Water: It's the most important part of a marathon. And so many times there isn't enough.

— FRED LEBOW

Marathon training is no great mystery. Don't throw your current training out the window in search of that "magic" marathon program.

— GRETE WAITZ

[The marathon is] kind of like the Ph.D. of public fitness accomplishments. There are very few times as an adult that you can go out and do something that's authentically difficult and be publicly lauded for it.

— MARCY IN CATE TERWILLIGER'S "MARATHON WOMAN"

One of the scariest things about running a marathon for the first time isn't the distance, the muscle pain, the chafing, or the blisters. It's not knowing what's going to happen.

— *RUNNER'S WORLD UK*

The standard prayer to St. Michael is, "St. Michael the Archangel, defend us on the day of battle, be our protection against the wickedness and snares of the devil." For me, marathon day is a battle and the last six miles are where the devil lays his snares and I ask St. Michael to help me out.

— LARRY SMITH

I've dropped out of many marathons. I'm not proud of it. I feel terrible dropping out, but if I have to do it, I do. It's part of the game, and often gives you the impetus to do better in the future.

— FRED LEBOW

I tend to run better if I put in very high mileage the week *before* I start my four-day countdown.

— BILL RODGERS ON PREPARING FOR A MARATHON

It's a poor man's race. You don't have to go to college or belong to any club, and there's nothing in it but a medal and a cup if you win. And yet they've been running this race for over forty years. There have been marathons ever since the Greeks defeated the Persians.

— KAY REYNOLDS IN GEORGE HARMON COXE'S "SEE HOW THEY RUN"

I am told there is a hill, but I didn't find it.

— FATUMA ROBA, AFTER WINNING THE BOSTON MARATHON

Almost every first-time marathoner says the same thing at the finish line: "Never again."

— BOB GLOVER, *THE RUNNER'S HANDBOOK*

If you can't stay patient and hold your body back, you are going to get in trouble and suffer later. It's also hard because you know you're at the beginning of a long journey.

— RYAN HALL

Those long runs cleanse my system, physically and mentally.

— JOAN BENOIT SAMUELSON

It is true that speed kills. In distance running, it kills anyone who does not have it.

— BROOKS JOHNSON

—⇒◆⇐—

There is the truth about the marathon and very few of you have written the truth. Even if I explain to you, you'll never understand it, you're outside of it.

— DOUGLAS WAKIIHURI, SPEAKING TO JOURNALISTS

—⇒◆⇐—

Baby boomers in general and boomer distance runners in particular were heirs both to the warrior mentality of their World War II-veteran fathers and the new consciousness of the 1960s and '70s. Both ways of thinking were essentially idealistic and challenged us to adopt causes greater than ourselves. The marathon served as an ideal outlet for both types of energy.

— TOM DERDERIAN

—⇒◆⇐—

I still think the marathon is easy, if you are mentally and physically prepared for it.

— STEVE JONES

———◆———

At mile 80, it's not all that great, but you live through it and then fondly recall how good it was.

— TIM TWIETMEYER, WINNER OF FIVE 100-MILE WESTERN STATES ENDURANCE RUNS

———◆———

Marathons are extraordinarily difficult, but if you've got the training under your belt, and if you can run smart, the races take care of themselves.

— DEENA KASTOR, FIRST AMERICAN WOMAN TO RUN A MARATHON UNDER 2:20

———◆———

I definitely want to show how beautiful the marathon can be. I am the opponent of all those who find the marathon bad: the psychologists, the physiologists, the doubters. I make the marathon beautiful for myself and for others. That's why I'm here.

— UTA PIPPIG

I have been asked everywhere I go: Why do people run the marathon? Sure, there is a sense of status we gain among our peers. But I think the real reasons are more personal. I think it is because we need to test our physical, emotional, or creative abilities.

— FRED LEBOW

If people were possessed by reason, running marathons would not work. But we are not creatures of reason. We are creatures of passion.

— NOEL CARROLL

It is a sublime thing to suffer and be stronger.

— HENRY WADSWORTH LONGFELLOW

I felt like I played in a very rough football game with no hitting above the waist.

— ALAN PAGE, FORMER NFL PLAYER

You can actually suffer a little bit more going slowly than when you're going really fast. A faster marathon might even be easier than a slow one, in terms of what it takes out of you mentally.

— FRANK SHORTER

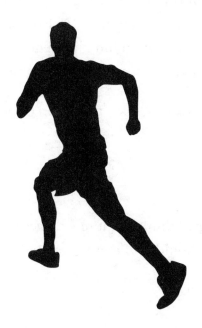

Even today, twenty-one years later, I still get chills when I remember [the roar of the crowd at the Boston Marathon in 1982]. It echoed and reverberated into this deafening, almost palpable wall of sound. It was very powerful. It sounded almost holy.

— JOHN LODWICK

As he staggered, half-blind in the dim light, to the foot of the hill, he thought of the Athenian runner finishing the first Marathon and, as he collapsed, crying, "Rejoice, we conquer!" Nilson realized how much that image, those words had been with him, influencing him all his life. They heartened him now, sealed the sense of meaning in him.

— HARRY SYLVESTER, "GOING TO RUN ALL NIGHT"

At the two-thirds mark, I think of those who are still with me. Who might make a break? Should I? Then I give it all I've got.

— IBRAHIM HUSSEIN

Being able to run fast means nothing, if you haven't trained your body to throw in a 4:40 mile at mile 25.

— RYAN LAMPPA

I'm never going to run this again.

> — GRETE WAITZ, AFTER WINNING HER FIRST OF NINE NEW YORK CITY
> MARATHONS

———◆◆◆———

The marathon can humble you.

> — BILL RODGERS

———◆◆◆———

I can't accept this marathon business: who wants to run 26 miles and 385 yards, in a competitive race? Jane does. For the last three months at least our lives have been taken over by those 26 miles, what we eat, what we do, where we go, and I have learned to hate every one of them.

> — SARA MAITLAND, "THE LOVELINESS OF THE LONG-DISTANCE
> RUNNER"

———◆◆◆———

In this mechanized society of ours, marathoners want to assert their independence and affirm their individuality more than ever. Call it humanism, call it health, call it folly. Some are Lancelots, some are Don Quixotes. All are noble.

— ERICH SEGAL

The marathon is like a bullfight . . . there are two ways to win. There's the easy way if all you care about is winning. You hang back and risk nothing. Then kick back and try to nip the leaders at the end. Or you can push, challenge the others, make it an exciting race, risking everything.

— ALBERTO SALAZAR

Look at me: a natural distance runner, wiry and muscular, trained down to gristle. We are the *infantry* of running. Your four-forty and eight-eighty men, these are your cavalry. The sprinters are your shock troops, your commandos.

— JOHN L. PARKER, JR., *ONCE A RUNNER*

When I knew I was going to win in 2004, I still felt awful. The last mile, I was just managing how much I was going to die.

> — ALAN CULPEPPER, WINNER OF THE 2004 U.S. OLYMPIC MARATHON TRIALS

I am too tired even to be happy.

> — GELINDO BORDIN, AFTER WINNING THE MARATHON AT THE HELSINKI OLYMPICS

The Boston Marathon has had more to do with liberating and promoting women's marathoning than any other race in the world.

> — JOE HENDERSON

For most runners, the marathon is like rolling dice.

— BOB SEVENE

———

Get going. Get up and walk if you have to, but finish the damned race.

— RON HILL TO JEROME DRAYTON DURING THE 1970 BOSTON
    MARATHON

———

The New York Marathon: a fantastic event.

— POPE JOHN PAUL II, 1982

———

The starting line of the New York City marathon is kind of a giant time
bomb behind you about to go off.

— BILL RODGERS

———

When I came to New York in 1978, I was a full-time school teacher and track runner, and determined to retire from competitive running. But winning the New York City Marathon kept me running for another decade.

— Grete Waitz

Marathoning is like cutting yourself unexpectedly. You dip into the pain so gradually that the damage is done before you are aware of it. Unfortunately, when awareness comes, it is excruciating.

— John Farrington

I just run as hard as I can for twenty miles, and then race.

— Steve Jones

Running cross-country is the closest man will ever get to flying.

— JOSEPH VANDERSTEL

The freedom of cross-country is so primitive. It's woman versus nature.

— LYNN JENNINGS

I was running to catch a train when one of my teachers saw me. He thought I was fast, timed me, and later gave me my first instructions in sprinting. I happened to be in the right place at the right time.

— ELIZABETH ROBINSON SCHWARTZ

The marathon is the focal point of all that has gone before and all that will come afterward.

— GEORGE SHEEHAN

Road racing is rock 'n roll; track is Carnegie Hall.

— MARTY LIQUORI

If you are going to do a marathon, decide what drink you are going to use way ahead of time, and use it in your long training runs.

— PRISCILLA WELCH ON ENERGY DRINKS

[T]he Médoc Marathon serves wine at its water stops. First prize is the winner's weight in grand crus.

— BENJAMIN CHEEVER, *STRIDES*

Cross-country was the earliest form of distance running and remains the most pristine, a race of athletes against the environment—often a twisting, hilly, even muddy environment. On a late October morning, a frost may cover the grass, so the runners make a crunching sound as they go through their warmup paces.

— AMBY BURFOOT, *THE RUNNER'S GUIDE TO THE MEANING OF LIFE*

Buzz [my dog] has reduced my range. Running safely with him means using fewer and shorter routes, with multiple laps per day or multiple returns there per week. Neither of us minds repeating ourselves. This is what runners do.

— JOE HENDERSON

Any idiot can run a marathon. It takes a special kind of idiot to run an ultramarathon.

— ALAN CABELLY

Training to run 100 miles is like training to get hit by a truck.

— LUIS ESCOBAR

If you feel good while running the Western States 100-mile Endurance Run, don't worry. You'll get over it.

GENE THIBEAULT

The race continued as I hammered up the trail, passing rocks and trees as if they were standing still.

— RED FISHER, ON HIS WASATCH FRONT 100 IN 1986

Surprisingly, the "idea" of running a hundred miles didn't frighten me. Instead, it awakened in me a curiosity, a wonder in myself, my ability, my strength, both physical and mental, and a quiet want. . . . I simply let it live inside me for a while, months, a year, two years, until I felt it coming out as stronger than just a murmur.

— KRIS WHORTON

If God invented marathons to keep people from doing anything more stupid, the triathlon must have taken Him completely by surprise.

— P. Z. PEARCE

The first fifty miles are run with the legs, the second fifty with the mind.

— ANONYMOUS

If you have a weak spot, the marathon will let you know.

— FRANK SHORTER

When you run there are no mistakes, only lessons. The art and science of ultra-running is a process of trial, error and experimentation. The failed experiments are as much a part of the process as the combination that ultimately works.

— KEITH PIPPIN

I really like cross-country. You're one with the mud.

— LYNN JENNINGS

I often leave my trusty routes through the country woods to explore new areas. Where does that road lead to? What is at the top of that hill?

— BOB GLOVER, *THE RUNNER'S HANDBOOK*

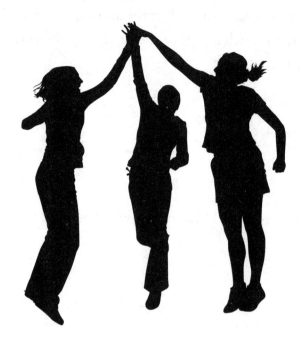

It's probably the toughest distance race in the world to win. World class runners from 1500m to the marathon contest it and instead of just three runners from each country, like in the Olympics or World Championships, in the senior men's race there are nine.

— PAUL TERGAT OF KENYA ON THE IAAF WORLD CROSS COUNTRY
CHAMPIONSHIPS

The marathon is charismatic. It has everything. It has drama. It has competition. It has camaraderie. It has heroism.

— FRED LEBOW

Run too far and the body doesn't want to stop.

— RICHARD CHRISTIAN MATHESON, "THIRD WIND"

The marathon is my benchmark. It is the status symbol in my community, the running community.

— GEORGE SHEEHAN

I am not entirely happy about the popularity of the marathon. Too many runners feel an obligation to run it. It is as though they cannot feel they are serious runners until they have met the challenge of the marathon.

— MARC BLOOM, *THE RUNNER'S BIBLE*

There's a park across the street from the house where I grew up. It took me a while to work up to running "all the way around the park." When I finally did, it was a really big deal. I ran all the way around the park! "You did what? All the way around? My goodness!" Everyone in my family was impressed. I had to lie down for the rest of the day. I measured it later—nine-tenths of a mile.

— Tish Hamilton, executive editor at *Runner's World*

I like hills because you can see the top. I know that sounds glib, but you know that the hill is not going to keep appearing; it's there and once you get to the top, it's behind you, and you feel as though you have conquered something.

— Rob de Castella

I found [sneakers] uncomfortable and after that I decided to continue running barefoot because I found it more comfortable. I felt in touch with what was happening—I could actually feel the track.

— ZOLA BUDD

On that day, we seemed to achieve what generations of politicians and philosophers have failed to do. With nothing more than our running shoes, we accomplished what all the wars and weapons have failed to do. We were, for a few hours anyway, a community of people whose sameness was more important than our differences.

— JOHN BINGHAM ON THE NEW YORK CITY MARATHON

A good hill definitely levels the playing field for a lot of runners, which means more of us not only will run closer together, but we will get a quality workout that would not be the same otherwise.

— "THE RAGE" ON BEATING YOUR BUDDIES

In an ultra you should eat like a horse, drink like a fish, and run like a turtle.

— ANONYMOUS

I was out training one black night when I heard a noise. I turned around and saw a leopard. I threw some stones at him and he went away, so I went on my way.

— FILBERT BAYI ON RUNNING IN HIS NATIVE TANZANIA

Running cross country is the closest man will ever get to flying.

— JOSEPH VANDERSTEL

All men may not be brothers, but that's the way it feels after a marathon. . . . You feel—you can't help but feel—that you all understand each other.

— BENJAMIN CHEEVER, *STRIDES*

The greatest treadmill running song, of course, is "Black Dog" from *Led Zeppelin IV*.

— PETE PFITZINGER

I never met a hill I couldn't walk.

— LARRY STICE

Most often . . . the women who saw me looked stunned; they didn't know how to react. . . . I wanted to say, "Yes, it's eighteen miles and I've run that far, and I will go twenty-six. Women *can* do this."

— KATHRINE SWITZER ON RUNNING MARATHONS

The other day I had a running scene, and I had two hours until my next scene. Instead of going back to the trailer, I kept on running for an hour.

— MIA MAESTRO, ACTRESS

You could go in any direction, fast or slow as you wanted, seeking out new sights just on the strength of your own feet and the courage of your lungs.

— JESSE OWENS

The start of a World Cross Country event is like riding a horse in the middle of a buffalo stampede. It's a thrill if you keep up, but one slip and you're nothing but hoof prints.

— ED EYESTONE

My introduction to track racing was through the background of cross country running, which is not a sport perhaps as popular in America as it is in England.

— ROGER BANNISTER

My dad was working out on the treadmill when Governor Bush called and officially asked him to be his running mate.

— MARY CHENEY

I love running cross country . . . on a track, I feel like a hamster.

— ROBIN WILLIAMS

I've always liked hills. I see a challenge, a goal, and I feel instantly galvanized to achieve the goal.

— AMBY BURFOOT, *THE RUNNER'S GUIDE TO THE MEANING OF LIFE*

A marathon is like life with its ups and downs, but once you've done it you feel that you can do anything.

— ANONYMOUS

When you run a marathon, you mean it. We're built for running. We dream of flying. For now, though, we're built to run.

— BENJAMIN CHEEVER, *STRIDES*

To describe the agony of a marathon to someone who's never run it is like trying to explain color to someone who was born blind.

— JEROME DRAYTON

Marathon running is a terrible experience: monotonous, heavy, and exhausting.

— VEIKKO KARVONEN, 1954 EUROPE AND BOSTON MARATHON CHAMPION

The standard prayer to St. Michael is, "St. Michael the Archangel, defend us on the day of battle, be our protection agains the wickedness and snares of the devil." For me, marathon day is a battle and the last six miles are where the devil lays his snares and I ask St. Michael to help me out.

— LARRY SMITH

You have to forget your last marathon before you try another. Your mind can't know what's coming.

— ANONYMOUS

———◆———

I did philosophy from miles five to eleven, trying to form one discriminating sentence about Socrates, Kant, Spinoza, Kierkegaard, whomever. When I came to the authors of *How to Be Your Own Best Friend*, I knew my mind was wandering and let go of systematizing.

— MAX APPLE, "CARBO-LOADING"

———◆———

I once ran thirty-one miles and after that there was nothing in the world I thought I couldn't do.

— KATHRINE SWITZER

———◆———

There is reason for viewing with considerable apprehension the sudden popularity of the so-called Marathon race. . . . It is only exceptional men who can safely undertake the running of twenty-six miles, and even for them the safety is comparative rather than absolute.

— *THE NEW YORK TIMES*, FEBRUARY 24, 1909

The long race is there always, as a sort of platform on which to evaluate, and sometimes alter your life.

— BENJAMIN CHEEVER, *STRIDES*

The natural urge when running a distance is to push harder and finish sooner—to race against time. Every second behind a deadline is a little defeat.

— JOE HENDERSON

I thought about running a marathon a long time ago, but I'm just not a runner.

— SHANNON MILLER

———◆———

After nine miles when I made my initial surge, I focused on running each of the next 5K segments as fast and relaxed as I could.

— FRANK SHORTER

———◆———

Men, today we die a little.

— EMIL ZATOPEK AT THE START OF THE OLYMPIC MARATHON

———◆———

[The marathon is] kind of like the Ph.D. of public fitness accomplishments. There are very few times as an adult that you can go out and do something that's authentically difficult and be publicly lauded for it.

— Marcy in Cate Terwilliger's "Marathon Woman"

When I'm training for a marathon, I soak in a hot tub every day, and get a weekly masssage.

— Anne Marie Lauck

And this long-distance running lark is the best of all, because it makes me think so good that I learn things even better than when I'm on my bed at night.

— Alan Sillitoe in "The Loneliness of Long-Distance Running"

A man starts on a track fancying he is cut out for a sprinter, and sticks to short work without ever trying his powers at anything else, until one day it comes to him . . . that longer journeys would suit him better.

— HARRY ANDREWS

He was thinking: There is nothing like the Marathon. Just the figures alone mean something: 26 miles, 385 yards.

— JOHN L. PARKER, JR., *ONCE A RUNNER*

Marathons are great, particularly if you run one or two a year.

— AMBY BURFOOT, *THE RUNNER'S GUIDE TO THE MEANING OF LIFE*

The marathon is the ultimate endurance test. Oh, sure, some people sometimes go longer than that. But 26 miles 385 yards is where racing ends and where ludicrous extremes begin.

— JOE HENDERSON

The winners run at speeds equaled or surpassed by no more than a handful of runners ever in the world. As important for me was the fact that more than fifteen thousand people from sixty-eight countries compete in our race.

— FRED LEBOW, ORGANIZER OF THE NEW YORK CITY MARATHON

To understand the marathon is to run it a lot. . . . You can't really know it until you've felt the other side of it. That's the only way it's possible.

— BILL RODGERS

Certainly the personal aspect of long-distance running, where success rest with the individual rather than the team, is similar to boxing. Perhaps the violence of boxing, directed at another individual, is sublimated in running, becoming a different kind of aggression. Both sports definitely require coming to terms with personal suffering in pursuit of success.

— DON KARDONG

Only those who will risk going too far can possibly find out how far they can go.

— T.S. ELIOT

The word 'cannot' should be removed from the vocabulary of all marathoners.

— HAL HIGDON, *MARATHONING A TO Z*

Do most of us want life on the same calm level as a geometrical problem? Certainly, we want our pleasures more varied with mountains and valleys of emotional joy, and marathoning furnishes just that.

— CLARENCE DEMAR

Avoid running long distances on two consecutive days, unless you are training for a marathon, to give your body time to recover. Listen to your body and pace yourself accordingly.

— *THE U.S. NAVY SEAL GUIDE TO FITNESS AND NUTRITION*

I was condemned to run track, but I didn't like it. For me, going out on the weekends with Jock's runners and doing 20 to 25 miles around Jamaica Pond was fun. I looked forward to it all week.

—JOHN A. KELLEY

To the spectators, it's a freak show with legs; to the legitimate runners, it's a test of speed and endurance; and to the exhibitionists, it's a chance to be a screwball before a ready-made gallery.

— WILL CLONEY

[Y]ou have to respect the distance, which is often said about marathons but applies equally to all distance running.

— AMBY BURFOOT, *THE RUNNER'S GUIDE TO THE MEANING OF LIFE*

After every experience, it's natural to reflect that you might have done better. Only after a marathon can I say I have given everything.

— KENNY MOORE

I wanted to try a marathon.

— GRETE WAITZ, WHEN ASKED WHY SHE HAD COME TO HER FIST NEW YORK CITY MARATHON

CHAPTER FIFTEEN

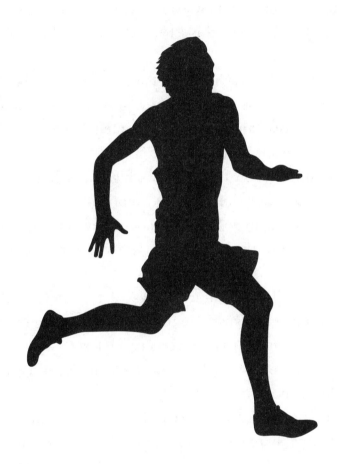

Long may you run

Finish Line

Each morning when we are at our winter home in Ponte Vedra Beach, Florida, I purchase the local newspaper, which includes a schedule of tides—high and low. I check this schedule daily. My life revolves around it. I run each day at low tide.

Low tide is when the beach is widest and flattest, thus, best for running. At high tide, the beach all but vanishes. Only a tiny slab of shore remains between ocean and houses. It is slanted, loose, often encrusted with shells and difficult for running.

Each day brings two low tides and two high tides, but not always at the same times. Low tide shifts forward approximately an hour each day, moving from morning to noon to afternoon to evening over a period of time. Thus, to know the best times to run, checking the schedule becomes essential.

As a committed, lifetime runner, I always have enjoyed running in scenic areas: through the woods, in the mountains, along the beach. But as that runner, I often ran past the scenery too fast to see it. Now as I have aged, I also have slowed. This low tide in my life finally has allowed me to slow down and, in effect, sniff the flowers.

Illness or injuries sometimes force runners into low tides, when we must modify activities to recover for high tides to come. Philosophers and physiologists might even argue over whether low and high tides represent low and high points in our lives. They could be either or both. They might be the opposite. More important, they represent change.

As a runner whose fastest days have passed, I may be at the point of low tide in my life. But it remains a very good time to run.

I've covered myriad teams where the fourth quarterback or third-string point guard is barely a part of things; where other players look down on him as inferior. There is a communal bond among harriers that I've yet to discover in another sport. Doing it *is* good enough in running. . .

  — Jeff Pearlman, "Heady Days: How a Lousy Collegiate
    Runner Eventually Made It to the Top"

Running has never failed to give me great end results, and that's why I keep coming back for more!

  — Sasha Azevedo

Running is a big question mark that's there each and every day. It asks you, "Are you going to be a wimp or are you going to be strong today?"

  — Peter Maher

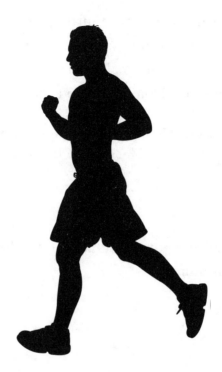

I never thought I'd have such a luxurious life. A healthy husband . . .
beautiful little girl . . . Jacuzzi and beer and fruit bowl and Beethoven
and Mendelssohn and running . . . Running is the best thing.

— MIKI GORMAN

[T]he effects of running are not extraordinary at all . . . It is the other states . . . that are peculiar, for they are an abnegation of the way you and I are supposed to feel. As runners, I think we reach directly back along the endless chain of history.

— James W. Fixx, *The Complete Book of Running*

Life is short. Running makes it seem longer.

— Baron Hansen

We run because it makes us feel like winners, no matter how slow or how fast we go.

— Florence Griffith Joyner and John Hanc, *Running for Dummies*

My feeling is that any day I am too busy to run is a day that I am too busy.

— JOHN BRYANT

I am already preparing for the day when I can't run at the top. Maybe I'll do more business, or just become a jogger.

— HAILE GEBRSELASSIE

The woods are lovely dark and deep.
But I have promises to keep,
And miles to go before I sleep,
And miles to go before I sleep.

— ROBERT FROST, "STOPPING BY WOODS ON A SNOWY EVENING"

Great is the victory, but the friendship of all is greater.

— Emil Zatopek

⟞⟞◆⟝⟝

It should make us proud to know we are part of a running lineage that stretches back from the original Olympic Games in 776 BC to this very moment.

— Michael Sandrock

⟞⟞◆⟝⟝

As I have aged, my running times and goals have changed, and so have my inspirations. I used to idolize the Olympic greats—the Paavo Nurmis, the Emil Zatopeks, the Abebe Bikilas, the Frank Shorters. Now I have a different hero—"Old John" Kelley, who has run the Boston Marathon sixty times.

— Amby Burfoot

⟞⟞◆⟝⟝

Vary your training, your running partners, and your environment. Only your imagination limits the ways you can spice up your running routine.

— Bob Glover, *The Runner's Handbook*

The secret shared by women runners: running is not just physical exercise but a spiritual, mental, and emotional journey.

— *Runner's Gazette*

Don't worry, everyone slows over time and I recall running slower at forty-three than at forty.

— Bill Rodgers

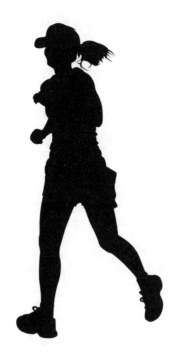

Just like I hope to be a mother the rest of my life, I hope to be a runner the rest of my life.

— JOAN BENOIT SAMUELSON

I plan to be running as long as I can and have no plans to stop.

— FRANK SHORTER

As he swept forward in line with the others a controlled jubilation came over him. Christ, I'm full of running! he thought. I'm absolutely full of running.

— VICTOR PRICE, "THE OTHER KINGDOM"

As we run, we become.

— AMBY BURFOOT, *THE RUNNER'S GUIDE TO THE MEANING OF LIFE*

The true runner is a very fortunate person. He has found something in him that is just perfect.

— GEORGE SHEEHAN

Tears streamed down my face as I crossed the finish line. I was a new person, a runner.

— THOMAS KING

Stay hungry and excited about what you are doing. It won't be forever and ever, because there will be a time when you want to bail out, because you want to do other things.

— PRISCILLA WELCH

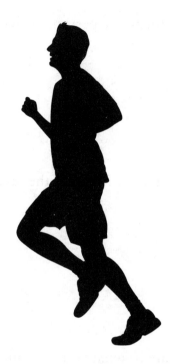

As every runner knows, running is about more than just putting one foot in front of the other; it is about our lifestyle and who we are.

— JOAN BENOIT SAMUELSON

I've had my fair share of being dismissed. But I'm only about to turn thirty. And when I finish running, I'm going to be a dangerous woman.

— CATHY FREEMAN

The old man asked me what I was running from. I was in full stride so I couldn't slow down to answer him. I could only hope that the wind carried my correction of "running toward" to his ears.

— NANCY LaMAR RODGERS

[E]ven when I'm eighty, I want to be one of the top three eighty-year-olds at the local races.

— STEVE STOVALL

Running has gone beyond fitness. The jogging movement, which began as a pursuit of health, has become an experiential quest.

— GEORGE SHEEHAN

You should not be flying down the home straight. Most of your efforts should have been put forth earlier.

— JOHN TREACY

In my mind, I'm still young. When I go to the starting line, I still perceive myself as racing in the open division.

— FRANCIE LARRIEU SMITH

My final and favorite ritual is the one I perform when I finish [a marathon]. As soon as I get home I take a long hot bath and drink cold beer in the tub. Then I lie on the bed and drink more beer, eat pretzels, and watch a videotape of the race.

— LARRY SMITH

Time doesn't stand still, and you don't stand still. Things change within yourself, within your life, and within your sport.

— PRISCILLA WELCH

Wisely and slow. They stumble that run fast.

— SHAKESPEARE, *ROMEO AND JULIET*

I've run a lot of miles over the years, some fast and some not so fast.

— ALBERTO SALAZAR

——◆——

Love yourself, for who and what you are; protect your dream and develop your talent to the fullest extent.

— JOAN BENOIT SAMUELSON

——◆——

Last is just the slowest winner.

— C. HUNTER BOYD

——◆——

Once you are a runner, it's always there in the back of your head.

— BILL RODGERS

——◆——

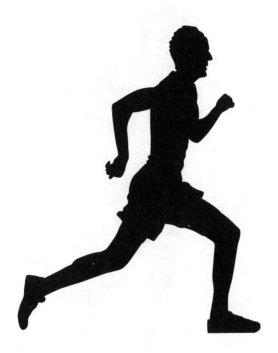

The more I run, the more I want to run, and the more I live a life conditioned and influenced and fashioned by my running. And the more I run, the more certain I am that I am heading for my real goal: to become the person I am.

— GEORGE SHEEHAN

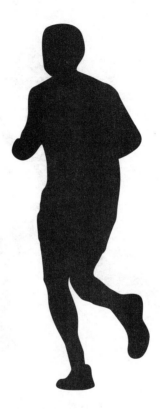

It's about time to stop; though don't think I'm not still running, because I am, one way or another.

— ALAN SILLITOE, "THE LONELINESS OF THE LONG-DISTANCE RUNNER"

Pray be always in motion.

— PHILIP DORMER STANHOPE CHESTERFIELD

In the longest run of all, your life, you're going to be a winner.

— AMBY BURFOOT, *THE PRINCIPLES OF RUNNING*

Keeping my eye on today is about all I'm capable of. And today, I think I'll go for a run.

— JOHN BINGHAM, "BACK TO THE FUTURE," *RUNNERS WORLD*

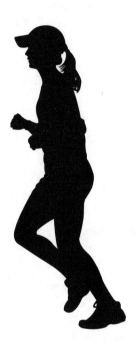

A comedian once claimed that all running does is to allow you to die in good health. Okay, I'll buy that.

— HAL HIGDON

Remember that if you don't go to the starting line, you will never view the whole course with all its possibilities. And you will certainly never see the glories of the finish line.

— AMBY BURFOOT, *THE RUNNER'S GUIDE TO THE MEANING OF LIFE*

Often, the enjoyment is the training before and the memory after.

— DOUG KURTIS

If I am still standing at the end of the race, hit me with a board and knock me down, because that means I didn't run hard enough.

— STEVE JONES

Winning has nothing to do with racing. Most days don't have races anyway. Winning is about struggle and effort and optimism, and never, ever, ever giving up.

— AMBY BURFOOT, *THE RUNNER'S GUIDE TO THE MEANING OF LIFE*

———

These records are only borrowed, precious aspects of the sport, temporarily in one's keeping.

— SEBASTIAN COE

———

You finished a marathon and you believe, 'If I can do this, I can do anything.'

— GRETE WAITZ AND GLORIA AVERBUCH, *RUN YOUR FIRST MARATHON*

———

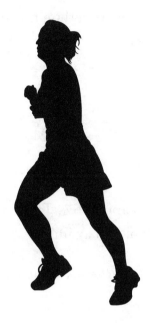

We walked through the parking lot. Neither of us said anything. We thought the world had ended.

— Anne Ryun, on husband Jim Ryun's retirement

Too many runners attempt the marathon much too early in their careers and then become ex-runners.

— ROBERT ESHICH

———❖———

I try to think of myself as an apple tree. Time is not linear, it moves in circles. Come spring, I will bloom again.

— AMBY BURFOOT, *THE RUNNER'S GUIDE TO THE MEANING OF LIFE*

———❖———

Sometimes I wonder whether I run high mileage so I can eat like this, or do I eat like this so I can run high mileage?

— BILL RODGERS, ON HIS FAVORITE SNACK OF MAYONNAISE AND CHOCOLATE CHIP COOKIES

———❖———

Rejoice. We conquer!

> — ATTRIBUTED TO THE ATHENIAN RUNNER WHO RAN FROM MARATHON
> ALL THE WAY TO ATHENS TO ANNOUNCE THE GREEK VICTORY OVER
> THE PERSIANS, AND THEN DIED.

THOSE QUOTED